Genes and the Biology of Cancer

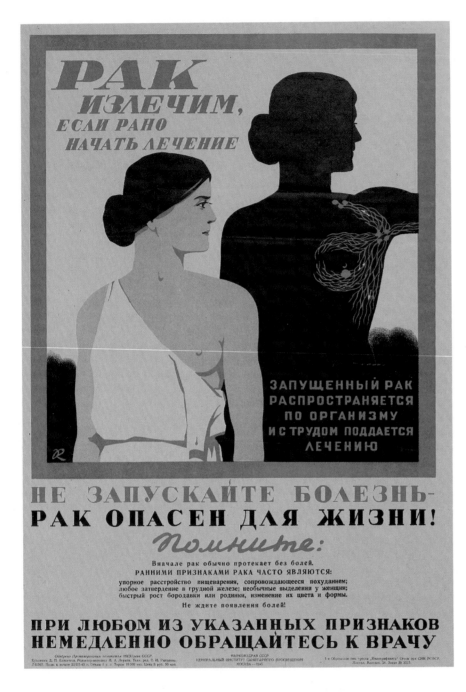

"Cancer can be cured,
if you start treating it
at an early stage."
A 1945 poster from
the Soviet Union.

GENES AND THE BIOLOGY OF CANCER

Harold Varmus
Robert A. Weinberg

**SCIENTIFIC
AMERICAN
LIBRARY**

A division of HPHLP
New York

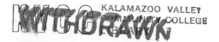

Library of Congress Cataloging-in-Publication Data

Varmus, Harold
    Genes and the biology of cancer / Harold Varmus,
Robert A. Weinberg.
      p. cm.
    Includes bibliographical references and index.
    ISBN 0-7167-5037-6
    1. Carcinogenesis. 2. Cancer cells. 3. Oncogenes. I. Weinberg,
Robert A. (Robert Allan), 1942– . II. Title.
    [DNLM: 1. Cell Transformation, Neoplastic. 2. Neoplasms—
etiology. 3. Oncogenes. QZ 202 V316c]
    RC268.5.V37 1993
    DNLM/DLC
    for Library of Congress   92-20554
                                            CIP

ISSN 1040-3213

Printed in the United States of America.

Scientific American Library
A division of HPHLP
New York

Distributed by W. H. Freeman and Company.
41 Madison Avenue, New York, New York 10010 and
20 Beaumont Street, Oxford OXI 2NQ, England

1 2 3 4 5 6 7 8 9 0 KP 9 9 8 7 6 5 4 3 2

This book is number 42 of a series.

CONTENTS

PREFACE

Recent discoveries have revolutionized the understanding of cancer. Our purpose in this book has been to show the motivated but non-expert reader how this understanding is structured and how these discoveries have emerged.

In large part, progress against cancer can be attributed to fundamental changes in the way organisms and diseases are now studied. Traditionally descriptive, biology has been transformed in the twentieth century into a science capable of explaining complex phenomena like cancer. This new power flows largely from a comprehension of genetics in molecular terms that descends both from Gregor Mendel's conception of the gene as the unit of heredity and from James D. Watson and Francis H. C. Crick's identification of genetic material as a double helix of DNA. But modern biology also depends upon biochemical methods for purifying molecules and characterizing enzymes; upon procedures for growing cells and viruses under controlled conditions; and upon physical techniques for describing molecules at the atomic level. All these approaches have had major roles in developing the radically new picture of cancer that we present in the pages that follow.

Even twenty years ago, ideas about the origins of cancer were obscure and conflicting. We now have a view of the genetic basis of cancer that, while still incomplete, is not only satisfyingly coherent but also remarkably precise in molecular detail. The essence of the story is disarmingly simple. Under normal conditions, the growth of each animal cell is exquisitely controlled—stimulated or retarded, according to need—by inherited (genetic) mechanisms. Cancer occurs when gene alterations (mutations) distort the normal controls in an individual cell, prompting it to inappropriate, ultimately invasive, growth. Such mutations can act directly, provoking cell growth, or indirectly, by impairing the means to restrict cell division.

The most profound revelations, however, are to be found in the details of the story. We now know most of the major components—the genes, proteins, and other molecules—that cells use to control their growth; the pathways through which these components interact; the exact form of the mutations that disrupt growth control; and the causes of some of these mutations. This knowledge leads inevitably and provocatively to questions about what can be done to avoid, forestall, or rectify the changes that contribute to cancer.

The story we have tried to tell is intricate, and our understanding has become remarkably sophisticated. If our ambition to convey the many complex facts about cancer has not unduly challenged our readers, we must thank the staff at W. H. Freeman and Company—especially Amy Johnson and Diana Siemens, who improved our prose and clarified our drawings, and Travis Amos, who made the pages beautiful by securing superb photographs. We also owe a great debt to the many colleagues who supplied illustrations, advice, and encouragement, and to those who made the discoveries that inspired us to write this book.

Harold Varmus
Robert A. Weinberg

July 1992

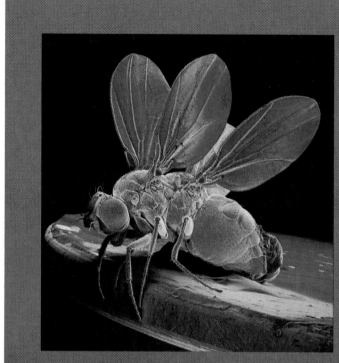

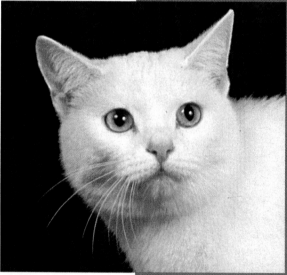

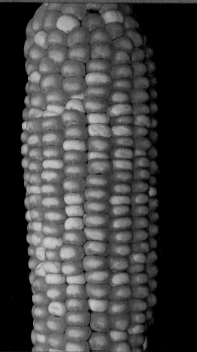

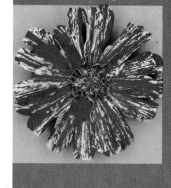

Mutations change individual organisms:
counterclockwise from top, a fruit fly's wings
(doubled), a cat's eyes, zinnia petals, and corn
kernels. Mutation, which drives evolutionary change,
also drives cancer.

1

GENES, CELLS, AND COMPLEX ORGANISMS

N ormal life processes are often directly illuminated by study of the abnormal. This book is another testament to the accuracy of that research adage; for the understanding it will record begins not with the beauties of living form, but with cancer, one of nature's aberrations. The fingers of a newborn child or the pattern of a butterfly's wing represent what we normally admire in biological systems: form; control; a unity of design and function that favors the survival of the organism. In cancer, all of these virtues are lost. Cancer cells divide without restraint, cross boundaries they were meant to respect, and fail to display the characteristics of the cell lineage from which they were derived. Yet it is from such cells, with their feared consequences for the organism, that biologists have learned many key mechanisms in the drama of normal growth and development. Conversely, to show why and how such mechanisms may fail—and may thereby initiate cancer—requires an initial review of our understanding of normal biological function; above all, of the general strategies that organisms use to govern their growth and differentiation.

All life on our planet depends upon one fundamental set of chemical components and processes. Living things are organized into functional units called cells; generate the same chemical, adenosine triphosphate (ATP), as their major source of energy; follow directions in a universal genetic code inherited in the same chemical form (deoxyribonucleic acid, or DNA); and, using nearly identical mechanisms, employ that code to make proteins and other components necessary for growth and, ultimately, the generation of new cells. (Viruses, whose credentials as living things remain controversial, conform to some but not all of these unifying features.) What is learned about one organism, then, may have significance for many others.

Although the universality of biological principles will be important at many stages of our story, a book about the molecular biology of cancer must emphasize at the outset a basic distinction that biologists make between simple, single-celled organisms, such as bacteria and yeast, and complex, multicelled organisms, such as plants, insects, and mammals. These complex organisms, composed of multiple tissues with different properties, must be endowed with genetic instructions for the growth

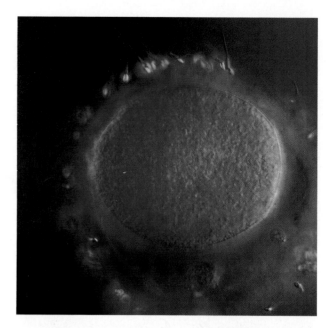

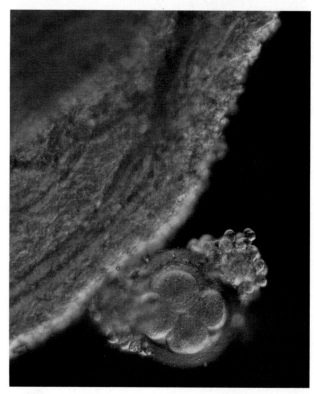

Sperm and egg unite (left); the single cell that results develops by successive divisions into a complex metazoan organism.

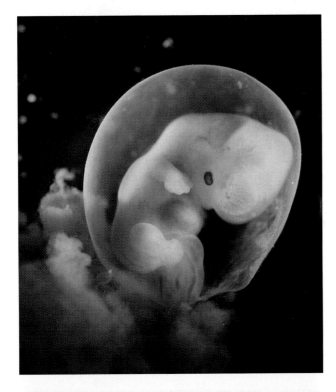

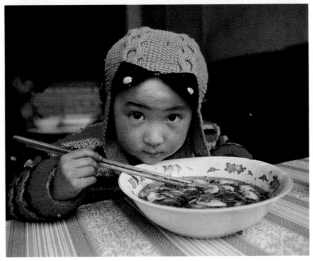

and maturation of many types of cells. When these instructions are distorted or fail, one possible result is the excessive growth of one cell type, often at the expense of others. In its most blatant form, the overgrowth invades locally and spreads to distant sites, finally killing the organism. When it affects human beings, we recognize this kind of derangement as cancer. The mechanisms underlying such events are the subject of this volume.

Disturbances of growth can and do occur in unicellular organisms, and they may be instructive for students of cancer. But true cancerous tumors (neoplasias) are found only in complex organisms and have been most fully characterized in animal species (metazoans). To understand neoplastic growth, therefore, it is necessary to establish some of the essential components of metazoans—the cellular units of which they are composed, the genetic instructions responsible for many of their properties, and the biochemical methods they use to put the instructions into action.

ESSENTIAL PROPERTIES OF CELLS

The basic unit of biological growth and development is the cell. Whether a living thing is undergoing normal development or control of growth has been lost, whether an organism is defined as a single cell or as an aggregate of many cells differing in appearance and function, each cell exhibits integrity of structure and a degree of autonomy.

At their peripheries, cells have physical boundaries that separate them from their envi-

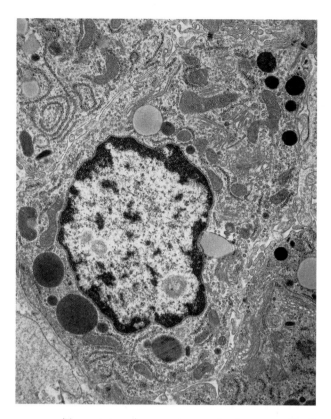

Transmission electron micrograph of an animal cell shows the large central nucleus and cytoplasmic molecular machines (organelles) that perform cell functions. Examples are the elongated mitochondria and the convoluted membranes of the Golgi apparatus and the endoplasmic reticulum.

Virtually all cells in a multicellular organism contain complete copies of the genetic instructions inherited from the organism's parents, to be passed in turn to its descendants. These instructions, in the form of long, two-stranded pieces of DNA, are present initially in a single cell, the fertilized egg—a precursor of the entire organism. This cell must undergo a large number of sequential divisions, each giving rise to two daughter cells, in order to produce the mature organism that, in humans, is composed of at least ten million million (10^{13}) cells. Following these inherited instructions, the cells not only multiply but also construct an imposing array of molecules that provide the cell architecture and perform the daily activities required both for survival and for specialized duties.

The complete set of genetic instructions in a cell is called its genome; the DNA molecules encoding the instructions are covered with proteins, together forming chromosomes. Cells are

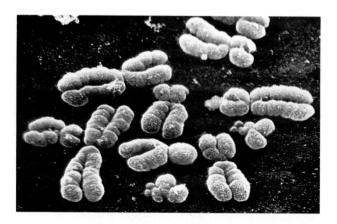

A scanning electron microscope yields a view of human chromosomes; the genome comprises 22 pairs, plus the sex chromosomes.

ronments. Animal cells are packaged in simple fatty membranes, but plants, bacteria, and yeast manufacture, in addition, less penetrable cell walls that lie just beyond the membranes. Inside these barriers all cells consist of protoplasm: a dense mixture of large molecules— nucleic acids (DNA and ribonucleic acid, or RNA), proteins, carbohydrates, and fats— suspended in salt water.

Germ Cells and Somatic Cells

Unlike single-celled organisms, multicellular animals normally cannot be regenerated from any single cell, even though most cells contain the organism's complete genome and may grow in the absence of their usual neighbors. Instead, the business of making a new organism has been assigned to specialized cells that are found exclusively in the testes (male) and the ovaries (female). These are called the germ cells. Ordinary body (somatic) cells of animals are diploid, endowed with two copies of all chromosomes, except for the sex chromosomes. (The sex chromosomes are usually named X and Y, whereas all the others, called autosomal chromosomes, are numbered.) Unlike these somatic cells, germ cells are able to reduce their number of chromosomes by one-half through a special process called meiosis. The products of meiosis are haploid cells called gametes—sperm in males, eggs in females—with one copy of each autosomal chromosome and one sex chromosome. Gametes combine to form a single cell (a fertilized egg, or zygote) with a complete and unique diploid set of chromosomes, half from each parent. By successive divisions, the zygote ultimately gives rise to the large number of descendants that form a complete organism. The cell divisions of these somatic (nongerm) cells through the process of mitosis ensure the transfer of the entire complement of chromosomes, both maternally and paternally derived, to progeny cells.

Any change in the genetic information carried by a germ cell will affect the genome of the resulting zygote and in turn all the cells of the new organism. Since that change is present in both somatic and germ cells, it may be transmitted to succeeding generations. As we shall see in later chapters, certain inherited variations in genetic information can place many somatic cells in human beings at high risk for the development of cancer. Genetic change that arises in a somatic cell, however, affects only that cell and any cells derived from it by further rounds of cell division in the maturing individual; such a change, since it is not present in the germ cells, cannot be transmitted to the individual's offspring.

assigned to one of two categories, depending upon whether they contain a nucleus to isolate their chromosomes from other parts of the protoplasm. In eukaryotic organisms (including plants, yeast, and animals) the genome is fragmented into linear chromosomes and enclosed by a second, internal membrane that separates it from most of the rest of the cell (its cytoplasm). In prokaryotic organisms such as bacteria, the genome is usually one large, circular chromosome that floats within the cell, unconstrained by a nuclear membrane.

Metazoan organisms have existed as interdependent communities of cells for over a billion years. Yet despite this long evolution, the individual cells within a metazoan continue to display a considerable degree of autonomy. Each cell maintains a distinctive identity and the ability to perform most or all of the functions found in free-living, unicellular organisms. Almost all cells within a complex animal are endowed with the ability to synthesize organized units of large molecules (organelles) that efficiently perform many tasks essential to the cell or to the multicellular partnership. The jobs assigned to these molecular machines include protein synthesis (performed by ribosomes), ingestion and secretion of macromolecules (endosomes, endoplasmic reticulum, Golgi apparatus), degradation of certain wastes (lysosomes), and generation of chemical energy (mitochondria). In addition, the cytoplasm, far from being an amorphous sludge, is organized into a fibrous network (the cytoskeleton) that gives shape to cells lacking cell walls, moves cells through their environment, and transports internal units within cells. Many cells are also equipped with machinery for enhancing their surroundings with a collection of fibers (the extracellular matrix) that promote cell adhesion, movement, and shape. Most cells, moreover, can duplicate all their constituents, including their chromosomal DNA, and divide, yielding two daughter cells.

The remarkable materials packaged within the cell membrane—a full set of genes, many enzymes, and organelles—provide a metazoan cell with its potential for autonomous behavior. Removed from its natural setting and placed in another hospitable context, such as a petri dish

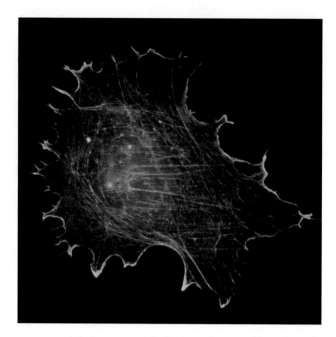

A light micrograph displays the actin fibers that help to form the cytoskeleton, essential to the architecture of an animal cell. In this human epithelial tissue cell from the lining of an organ, the actin matrix is dyed immunofluorescent orange.

supplied with nutrients and moisture, even a cell from a complex organism can retain the credentials of living things: the ability to grow and divide, to ingest and secrete, to build large molecules from small ones and degrade large ones to small. The perhaps unexpected autonomy of metazoan cells has both virtues and disadvantages. On the one hand, cells that can survive and multiply in a variety of contexts within the organism are free to move around, providing specialized functions throughout the body. On the other, cellular autonomy encompasses the potential for excessive growth, manifested ultimately as cancer.

Cellular Environments

Each cell in a complex organism, despite the remarkable autonomy we have emphasized so far, inhabits an environment—including extracellular fluids, dissolved chemicals, and insoluble fibers—that has been created by a wide variety of cells, both near and far. Even unicellular organisms possess devices (for example, sensors and propellers) for responding to changes in their surroundings, such as altered levels of nutrients or noxious substances. As might be expected from their need to intercommunicate, cells from metazoan organisms are especially well equipped in this respect. Such cells can both respond to and affect their environment in many ways, like individuals in a society. Cells in complex animals like humans are influenced by the nutrients, salts, and relative acidity of the fluids bathing them; by hormones secreted by distant organs; by factors produced by adjacent cells; and by the components of the extracellular matrix in which they reside.

Because cells can be removed from the normal environment in a tissue and grown in culture, a researcher can separate them from the normal array of signals that impinge on them and, in the confines of a petri dish, impose a new set of signals. Thus the timing of cell division, the direction of cell movement, and the execution of specialized cell functions can be manipulated by the experimenter, who can add or subtract components of the culture fluids, adjust the density and types of cells, or change the physical characteristics of the surface on which cells grow.

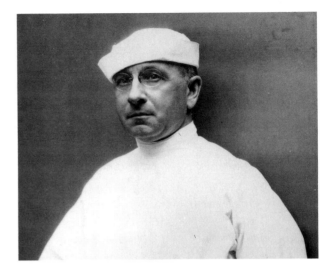

Alex Carrel, 1873–1944. Born in France, Carrel joined the Rockefeller Institute in 1906. He won a Nobel Prize in 1912 for research in vascular surgery and organ transplantation; in 1936 he and the aviator Charles A. Lindbergh invented a perfusion pump that they called an artificial heart. A pioneer in cell culture, Carrel kept cells from a chicken heart alive in his laboratory for 32 years.

Activities of Disrupted Cells

Cell biology focuses on the action of whole cells, but ultimately the behavior of each cell must be traced to the action of the multitude of molecules within it, the chemical reactions in which they participate, and the structures that they form. We are now in the realm of modern biochemistry and molecular biology, much of which is based upon the principle that many important components of cells—whether enzymes, organelles, or chromosomes

—may retain their essential structural and functional properties even after being removed from their usual intracellular contexts. Of course, once the integrity of the cell is violated, the orchestrated display of simultaneous functions that we call life is no longer possible. Disruption of the outer boundary of the cell—the membrane—will render the internal components unable to grow and divide, to move, or to respond to signals. Yet under appropriate conditions, many (but not all) of the individual processes essential to life can be continued in the material prepared from a disrupted cell: many cell proteins can still function as enzymes to catalyze certain chemical reactions; molecules containing genetic information may remain intact and may be manipulated to direct the synthesis of proteins; and multicomponent cellular machines, such as ribosomes and cell membranes, will continue to perform their normal tasks. Experimental success in isolating individual components and maintaining their activities after rupture of cells has been essential to the development of techniques that permit tinkering with—and promote an understanding of—fundamental cell activities, including many that are central to the problem of cancer.

THE GENETIC BLUEPRINT AND ITS VARIATIONS

Nowhere has this ability to dissect the essential ingredients of cells advanced our view of life processes more profoundly than with respect to the genetic blueprint. The blueprint, which contains the information necessary to make all the proteins involved in both normal cell growth and cancer, is laid out in the chromosomes that organisms inherit from their parents and individual cells acquire from their cellular precursors. The genetic instructions exist in the form of a double-stranded helix of DNA composed of four basic units, the nucleotides (or, more properly, deoxyribonucleotides), named after their bases: adenine, cytosine, guanine, and thymidine—abbreviated A, C, G, and T. The A's on one strand always pair with T's on the other; reciprocally, C's pair with G's. The information content of DNA is embodied in the sequential arrangement of the nucleotides. The same is true of the other major nucleic acid, RNA, whose bases are identical with those of DNA except that uracil (U) takes the place of thymidine. (Some viruses, unlike all other organisms, carry their genetic information in the form of RNA rather than DNA.)

If we could scan a DNA sequence from one end of a chromosome to the other, we would find instructions, or signals, that determine the precise chemical composition of many proteins. Closely associated with these protein coding sequences are regulatory sequences that determine when a protein will be made, and in what quantities. Together the protein coding and regulatory sequences comprise a gene. Most genes are about 10,000 to 100,000 nucleotides in length; about 5000 of them are arranged along the average human chromosome. Although the information for making any single protein is almost always encoded by a single gene, one gene may sometimes carry the information needed to make several related proteins.

Actual production of proteins occurs in the cytoplasm of the cell. Since the instructions for how to carry out this production are stored in the chromosomal DNA in the nucleus, an intermediary molecule—messenger RNA—must be synthesized to convey information from the nuclear storage repository to the cytoplasmic protein factory. The enzyme RNA polymerase transcribes the genetic information into an RNA copy from the nuclear DNA template. Because the protein-coding information is interrupted by irrelevant sequences (introns), the RNA must be edited (spliced) to remove the intron sequences and join the coding sequences (from exons). The messenger RNA that results from these transcription and processing events then moves to the cytoplasm, where it is used to generate protein.

This process, called translation, is accomplished by threading the messenger RNA through ribosomes, like a tape through the head of a tape player, to decode the information and assemble amino acids into chains.

Each adjacent group of three nucleotides (a codon) specifies the next amino acid to be linked to the growing protein chain; translation, in effect, reads codons as if they were words, calling out one of the 20 possible amino acids for specific addition to the protein under synthesis. The properties of each protein are determined by the sequence of amino acids used to construct it, and this sequence in turn is determined directly by the nucleotide sequence of the messenger RNA template.

REGULATION OF GENE EXPRESSION

Although a mammalian cell possesses the genetic instructions to make on the order of 50,000 to 100,000 different proteins, only a subset of those proteins, perhaps 10 to 20 percent, are found in any single cell. This obser-

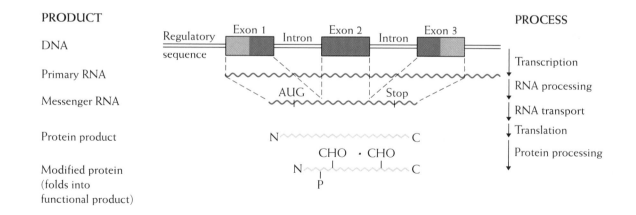

Gene transcription in a metazoan is initiated by a regulatory sequence of DNA nucleotides. After transcription into RNA, the genetic information is edited and spliced to omit the introns. Messenger RNA, transported out of the nucleus, is translated into protein on the cytoplasmic ribosomes.

vation introduces a new level of complexity into our understanding of genes, for it suggests that in each type of cell some genes are read out (by synthesis of messenger RNA molecules that, in turn, are used as templates to make diverse proteins), whereas other genes are silent (not read out). Moreover, different sets of genes are expressed in different types of cells, and among those genes that are read out (expressed), the outputs of gene products (proteins) can vary up to a millionfold. This means that in addition to the sequences that encode a protein, each gene must contain instructions that regulate production of the protein in correct amounts, at the correct times, for each cell type.

Gene expression can be regulated at several points. Most obvious and common are differences that result from the control of transcription: the amount of messenger RNA produced from a single gene can vary by many orders of magnitude. For example, the synthesis of messenger RNA for the protein component of hemoglobin occurs at extremely high rates in red-blood-cell precursors but at negligible levels in most other cells, even though they also carry copies of the gene for making hemoglobin. Later steps in the overall process of gene expression also afford points of control. The concentration of messenger RNA can be regulated by how fast it is synthesized in the nucleus; by its rate of transport to the ribosomes, where translation occurs; and by its relative ability to survive, once in the cytoplasm. If the messenger RNA is stable, it can be used repeatedly to make new protein chains; if quickly degraded, its capacity to direct protein synthesis will be correspondingly limited.

Still other constraints operate upon translation, influencing, for example, the likelihood that the ribosome factories will use a given messenger RNA molecule to make a protein. The long- or short-term stability of a newly synthesized protein can determine whether it will accumulate in a cell, and chemical modifications can influence its biological activity. Some proteins, for example, must have certain chemical groups—sugars, phosphates, or sulfates—attached to them in order to perform their normal functions; others must be broken apart (cleaved) at defined positions. The ability to make these modifications can create differences between cells as important as those achieved by different rates of RNA synthesis.

GENETIC VARIATION, MUTATION, AND VIRUSES

This information for regulating protein synthesis, encoded using the four "letters" of the DNA "alphabet," makes biological variability possible at levels from cell type through species. Even individual variability within a species may be ultimately traced to subtle differences in the structure of proteins or the programs that dictate their production.

Biological variability implies that the underlying genetic blueprint is enormously plastic. The information content of DNA can be altered dramatically by minute changes in the order of its nucleotides or by gross rearrangements of its sequences. In other words, the meaning carried by a gene can be affected by even the subtlest alteration of its text.

Such changes are caused by mutation, the process that continually introduces small or large variants into the genetic text from one generation to the next. Within a species, mutation leads to ever-increasing genetic diversity among its individual members; over evolutionary time periods, this diversity generates new species. The fact that each individual is built and behaves differently from all others within a species is thus attributable to the process of mutation.

Mutation thus drives evolutionary change. Those individuals lucky enough to inherit a particular, advantageous combination of mutant genes may be greatly favored in the struggle to survive and reproduce, passing their gene copies on to their descendants. But mutation is also the central force behind the process of cancer. Almost all cancers result from alterations of genes in somatic cells—mutations that affect a given cell and its descendants in an individual rather than every cell in an organism and its offspring.

How does mutation occur? In general, cells reproduce their genetic blueprints for transmission to daughter cells with astonishing fidelity; in the course of copying a few billion nucleotides (also termed bases), fewer than a hundred

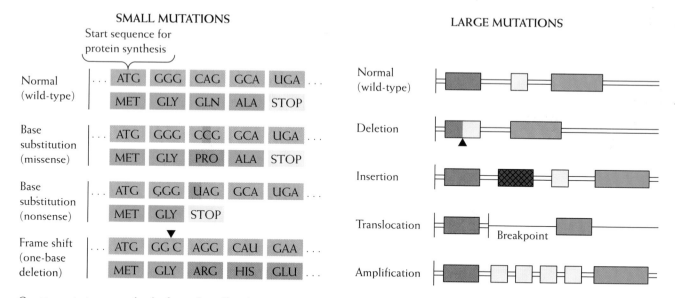

Genetic variation can take the form of small or large mutations in an organism's DNA, as the scheme above illustrates. Large mutations may involve the insertion of foreign, perhaps viral, genetic information (purple box) or the exchange of information by translocation between two chromosomes at a breakpoint. Small mutations result from changes in a single base (nucleotide) or codon (nucleotide triplet, dictating a particular amino acid in the protein product).

errors are likely to be made, most of them inconsequential. Even this low error frequency, however, means that each round of cell division is accomplished by genetic diversification that is potentially damaging. In fact, given the large number of cells in an adult human being, it is likely that each of an individual's tens of thousands of genes has experienced at least some damage in several or more somatic cells.

To produce genetic variations—mutations—DNA may be altered in a number of ways. In the simplest case, a single nucleotide (and ultimately its complementary nucleotide on the other strand of the double helix) is changed. Such base substitutions may have little or no impact (if, for example, they do not direct a corresponding change in protein sequence). Or they may have a variety of effects on gene function, changing signals for transcription, RNA processing, or translation. They may alter codons within protein coding sequences to conclude translation prematurely (nonsense mutation) or to incorporate a different amino acid (missense mutation). These changes are especially obvious when a critical amino acid in an important protein is replaced by an amino acid with different chemical properties. Sickle-cell anemia, a well-known example, is a disease caused by the inheritance of a base-substituting mutation that alters a single amino acid in one of the components of hemoglobin.

Other mutations are more complex, involving loss, duplication, or rearrangement of DNA. Deletions, for example, can range in size (and consequences) from a single nucleotide pair (which would drastically alter reading of the subsequent triplet codons) or a single codon (which would remove one amino acid from the normal protein product of a gene) to large expanses of a chromosome (perhaps eliminating multiple genes). Very large deletions, of course, are tolerated only if they do not incapacitate essential genes, or (in diploid cells, which contain paired chromosomes) if a normal gene is retained by the parallel chromosome. Common rearrangements other than deletions include exchanges of DNA between two chromosomes (translocations), inversions of DNA segments, and even the acquisition of genetic information from elsewhere by the insertion of DNA into a chromosome.

Such DNA insertions may be donated by other genes within the same cell or by viruses that have invaded the cell, carrying in foreign genetic sequences. Chromosomes of all organisms, including human beings, contain many kinds of semiautonomous units, generally a few hundred to a few thousand base pairs in length, called mobile genetic elements. Although their purposes and origins remain matters for speculation, it is well established that they are able to move within the genomes of their host cells, often while duplicating themselves. By jumping from one chromosomal site to another, a mobile DNA segment may disrupt and inactivate a gene into which it has inserted itself, or it may alter the gene's pattern of expression. Since mobile elements are so abundant in mammalian genomes, there has been considerable conjecture about the role their movements might play in the mutations that trigger cancer, but so far only sporadic evidence has been produced.

Viruses, then, can be the source of permanent genetic change in cells, by inserting their

Genotypes and Phenotypes

The study of genetics by Gregor Mendel and his many later disciples was initially stimulated by inherited changes in the appearance or behavior of organisms—the so-called phenotype. Various aspects of an organism's phenotype can be followed as markers for genes: the color of pea flowers, or mouse fur; the nutritional requirements of bacteria or yeast; certain diseases of human beings. Individual genes were originally defined by the phenotypic effects that they create. These days, variations in phenotype can often be traced to specific changes in the governing genes—that is, to mutations in their nucleotide sequence.

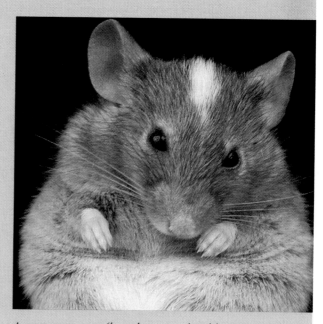

A mutant genotype (here, due to an altered kit gene) is reflected in the individual phenotype: a characteristic pigmentation pattern in mammals (the piebald trait).

This underlying genetic information is referred to as an organism's genotype.

The white spotting (piebald) trait characterized by an absence of hair pigment in specific places appears in mice or in human beings that inherit inactive mutant copies of the same gene, called kit. When a different kind of mutation makes the kit gene hyperactive, it contributes to the formation of a cancer cell (see Chapters 4 and 6). In these instances, the phenotype of the affected individual or cell provides a clue to the responsible genotype.

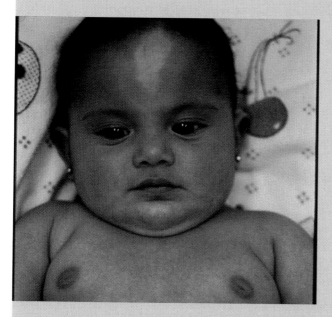

A human infant displays the piebald trait.

DNA into the chromosomes of cells they infect. One consequence of the addition of viral information may be a deregulation of the cell's growth, leading in turn to excessive proliferation; in this way viruses play an indisputably central role in the development of cancer in experimental animals and, sometimes, in human beings. The addition of viral DNA may cause deregulation because a chromosomal gene has been mutated thereby or because the virus has introduced a gene of its own, which then promotes inappropriate growth.

These facts run counter to common ideas about viruses, which normally do not establish long-term relationships with the cells they infect. Most of the disease-inducing viruses of humans, such as those that cause colds, polio, or encephalitis, seem to have the simple objective of taking over the reproductive machinery of an invaded cell in order to make many thousands of new virus particles; the commandeered cell is destroyed as a result. But several kinds of viruses occasionally, and even (in the case of retroviruses) routinely, deposit DNA copies of their genes in host chromosomes without killing the infected cell. Most of these viruses can cause cancer in animals or human beings. The viral cancer genes they introduce and the host-cell genes they mutate will be important subjects of subsequent chapters.

HOMOLOGS AND GENE FAMILIES

Many genes that were evolving in our ancestors a billion and more years ago persist in similar form in our genome today. Indeed, versions of such highly conserved genes are likely to be present in many (sometimes all) modern metazoans. Genes descended from a common ancestral gene are said to be homologs, even when the living organisms appear to be only distantly related. Conservation over vast evolutionary time periods implies that the gene is vital for organismic or cellular function, so any attempts by the mutational processes of evolution to tinker excessively with its basic content will result in disaster.

Biological research benefits profoundly from this circumstance. Certain genes and their

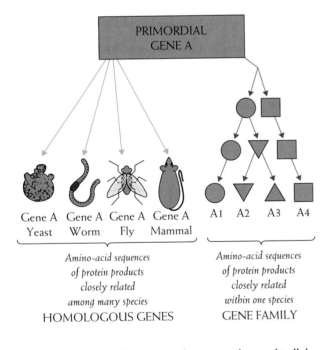

Amino-acid sequences of protein products closely related among many species
HOMOLOGOUS GENES

Amino-acid sequences of protein products closely related within one species
GENE FAMILY

A primordial gene may be conserved in multicellular organisms for more than a billion years, either as homologs among various species or as a varied gene family within a single species.

encoded proteins may be difficult to study in humans, but their homologs, having very similar functions, may be studied easily in mice, fruit flies, worms, or even yeast. Lessons learned in these organisms may then be transferable to our understanding of the human condition.

Within a given organism's genome, there are groups of genes that are clearly related to one another. In relatively simple ancestral organisms, a small number of genes encoded a correspondingly small number of proteins. Many of those genes have been duplicated and reduplicated as the simpler organisms evolved into more complex ones, creating families of closely related genes. Although basically similar in structure, the proteins encoded by the various members of a gene family may have taken on slightly different, specialized functions—for example, related proteins with similar enzymatic activities may be made in different cell types, where they act upon different target molecules.

THE CELL CYCLE AND CELL GROWTH

Of the many functions performed by individual cells, growth and division are the most germane to the problem of cancer. The normal generation of a multicellular organism depends completely upon these processes, which permit cells to undergo many rounds of duplication without loss of mass or genetic potential.

The entire sequence of events that produces two daughter cells more or less indistin-guishable from a parental eukaryotic cell is called the cell division cycle (or cell cycle). For a typical somatic cell from a vertebrate animal, the length of the cycle is generally between 12 and 24 hours, although it can be considerably shorter during development of the embryo. Two features are essential for successful execution of the cell cycle. First, the parental cell must grow large enough and produce enough of its staples to supply each of the two daughter cells with a full complement of ingredients, including DNA, RNA, proteins, organelles, membranes, salts, and fluids. Second, the cell must have the means to coordinate the intricate steps in the cell cycle with the production of cellular materials.

Careful observation of cells undergoing growth and division reveals that the cell cycle is choreographed with considerable precision. Two major events are especially easy to discern: the duplication of the cellular genome (the DNA synthesis or S phase) and the subsequent separation of the two equal portions, each destined for one of the daughter cells (the mitotic or M phase). M phase usually lasts 1 to 2 hours; S phase takes several hours. Between these two central phases there are two gaps, called G1 and G2, during which the cell synthesizes many of the building blocks it will need to proceed to the next phase. Thus, in the G1 gap the cell accumulates the enzymes needed to duplicate the genome and amasses the other ingredients required to supply the daughter cells with proper resources, permitting S phase to commence only after checkpoints have been passed. During the G2 gap, which follows S phase and precedes M phase, the cell prepares itself for mitosis and checks to be certain that DNA replication has been successfully completed. In short, the cell constantly monitors what it has accomplished before it commits itself to proceeding through the next critical step of its cycle.

During the several hours of S phase, the cell must make an accurate copy of all its DNA; in human cells this totals about three billion pairs of nucleotides, spread over 23 pairs of chromosomes. This duplication is achieved by using each strand in the double helix of parental DNA as a template for the synthesis of new strands by enzymes called DNA polymerases. By the end of S phase, every chromosome has yielded two daughter chromosomes, each of which carries a DNA double helix comprising an old strand (from the parental chromosome) and a new strand (manufactured by pairing complementary nucleotides to the design provided in the parental DNA strand). If all goes well, the cell generates two new double helices that are precise copies of one another and identical to the double helix present in the parental cell prior to synthesis.

M phase segregates the newly replicated chromosomes into appropriate portions of the enlarged parental cell so that it can be divided into two independent daughter cells in a fashion that guarantees equal allotment of the genetic blueprint to each. Prior to cell division, the duplicated chromosomes are aligned and redistributed to either side of the parental cell by a fibrous machine constructed by the mitotic cell. During this process, the nuclear membrane that normally segregates the chromosomes from the cytoplasm is broken down. Upon division into two daughter cells, each

proceeds to enclose its allotment of chromosomes within a new nuclear membrane.

How does a cell manage to choreograph these steps in precise order? Studies of a wide range of eukaryotic organisms including yeast, clams, frogs, and mammals reveal a remarkably similar plan, executed by modular components that experimenters can swap between organisms whose common ancestors existed more than a billion years ago. The exchangeability of parts shows that a master clocking mechanism governing the cell cycle developed long ago and has been preserved with great fidelity in all descendant organisms over more than a million millennia.

In this plan, complex events like DNA replication and chromosomal segregation are triggered by centralized chemical regulators that are able to recruit the many components required for S and M phases. Each of these master regulators is now known to be an enzyme that can efficiently modify a wide range of proteins. These cell cycle regulators—like many other influential proteins to be described in this book—are protein kinases, enzymes designed to transfer phosphate groups from ATP (adenosine triphosphate) molecules (the cellular energy source) to specified amino acids in certain target proteins. The result of this phosphorylation process—the presence of a newly attached phosphate group—causes the target protein to gain or lose a function: to assemble or disassemble in the case of a structure-building molecule; to turn a biochemical reaction on or off in the case of a catalytic enzyme. Because each kinase may modify a variety of proteins, it can elicit a wide range of responses in the cell simultaneously.

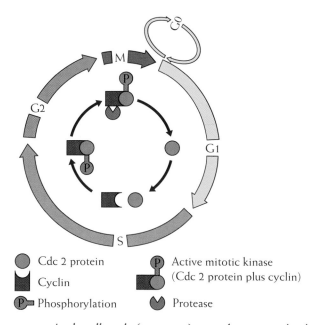

Cdc 2 protein

Cyclin

P— Phosphorylation

P Active mitotic kinase
(Cdc 2 protein plus cyclin)

Protease

As the cell cycle (outer ring) proceeds, it is regulated by the oscillation of cyclin protein, as the schematic inner ring suggests. During M phase, Cdc 2 protein bound to cyclin and suitably phosphorylated has an active mitotic kinase activity. When protease enzyme destroys cyclin, Cdc 2 protein is no longer activated, and the cell may enter G1 or rest in G0. When cyclin is again synthesized and accumulates, the Cdc 2 protein undergoes sequential phosphorylations and activation, leading again to M phase.

To avoid the chaos that would result from continual phosphorylation of their targets, the governing protein kinases must themselves be regulated. This happens in large part by the periodic rise and fall of another class of proteins called cyclins (the number of phosphates present on the protein kinases may also vary). Cyclins regulate kinase activity directly. The oscillation of cyclin concentrations imparts an autonomous quality to the cell cycle.

To prevent unremitting cell growth and division, cells traversing the cycle are equipped with important guidelines. It is as though each cell were an automobile traveling on a circular highway with signposts, barriers, and exits for delays, rest stops, and detours. For example, most cells are not committed to passage through the cell cycle until they have gone past physiological tollgates called start points. The presence of these points, commonly found near the start of S phase, suggests that the cell has delicate sensors that determine whether it is ready to carry out the complex events of that phase. Equally important, cells can exit the cell cycle in an interval that almost always follows M phase, by entering the rest stop called G0. Cells may remain quiescent in G0 for hours, days, or years.

Withdrawal from the cycling mode into G0 and return from G0 into the active G1 phase occur in response to environmental signals provided by general growth conditions (nutrients, temperature, salts) or by specific proteins, known as growth factors, that interact with designated receptors on the cell surface. These factors, their diverse roles in control of growth and differentiation, the mechanisms by which they stimulate growth, and their involvement in cancer will be described in detail in Chapter 6. But here we can already note that this choice between active cycling and G0 resting represents a most important decision point by which the numbers of cells in the body are controlled. Events that damage the cell's regulatory apparatus, trapping it in the active growth cycle, are critical initiators of the inappropriate growth of a cancer cell.

Development and Differentiation

A mature multicellular organism contains many kinds of cells, as judged by their appearance (morphology), the proteins they make, and their physiological functions. The more than 10^{13} cells in an adult human being are found in many different organs (such as the liver, brain, and skin); within each of these organs, there are a number of distinct tissues; and each tissue is composed of cells in different stages of development. As a result, more than 200 types of human cells can be accurately classified by morphological and functional criteria. Yet all are descended from a single fertilized egg, and virtually every cell is endowed with a complete, identical set of genetic instructions. (In mammals, mature red blood cells and platelets are exceptions, each lacking a nucleus and its DNA.) Because of this, each nucleated adult cell should have the potential to develop into many cell types. But it does not ordinarily display such potential, instead committing itself irrevocably to become one or another cell type and thus taking instruction from only a subset of the genes it carries in its nucleus.

When and how are such choices made? And what mechanisms are used to produce a cell that behaves in one way rather than another? During the early development of an embryo (three or four cell doublings after fertilization in mammals), individual cells begin to display specialized behavior and lose their ability to generate a complete organism. When this happens, these cells are said to have acquired a certain destiny, being slated to produce progeny that include some cell types but not others. The processes by which such destinies are fixed and then increasingly narrowed during later development—still poorly understood—are broadly termed differentiation. Some of the basic principles are known, however, and include mechanisms that often go awry in the generation of cancer cells.

The acquisition of specialized traits by a given metazoan cell depends critically upon its position in the developing embryo. Placement affects the signals that a cell receives from its neighbors, and these signals in turn affect which genes it reads out and so which proteins it produces. Such cells retain a full comple-

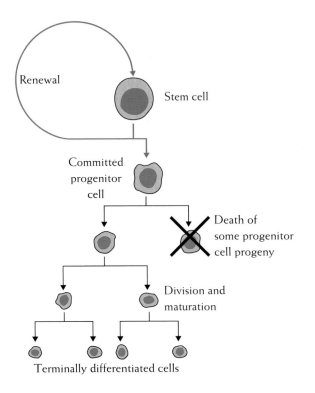

Stem-cell division may result in replication or differentiation along one of several pathways.

Model Systems for Developmental Biology

One of the central tasks of developmental biology is to identify the factors and genes used to communicate among cells in an embryo and control their destinies. This work is pursued in a variety of experimental systems, including several vertebrates (mice, chickens, frogs, and fish), insects (mainly the fruit fly *Drosophila melanogaster*), worms (principally the nematode *Caenorhabiditis elegans*), and even unicellular organisms (such as brewer's yeast or certain bacteria) that develop into specialized cells in response to environmental conditions.

Each of these organisms has its advantages. The unicellular organisms offer experimental speed and easy genetic manipulation. The *C. elegans* adult is simple enough to allow deduction of a complete lineage map of all its 1000 or so cells. (A lineage map is a chart of how each cell division leads in succession to all the cells in the fully developed adult.) *D. melanogaster*'s long history as an object of genetic study has generated a wealth of developmental mutants that illustrate how particular genes in normal or aberrant form regulate specific steps of embryologic development. And the vertebrate animals have body plans and developmental programs similar to those of human beings.

Two features of developmental biology make the study of these varied organisms of immense interest to anyone seeking to understand cancer. First, the biochemical mechanisms controlling development appear to be similar if not identical to those that govern cell growth and most often go awry in the making of a cancer cell. Second, the genes devoted to development and growth control in highly divergent organisms have proved to be so strongly conserved during evolution that it is possible to recognize members of the same gene family in yeast, worms, flies, and mammals. Thus the opportunities for understanding genes and proteins instrumental in human cancer are greatly enhanced by the study of development in more tractable organisms.

ment of genetic instructions, but the regulated use of subsets of genes allows them to take on the specialized patterns of behavior characteristic of tissues in mature organisms.

The nature of the cell-to-cell signals that govern developmental events provides yet another example of the extraordinary conservation of basic mechanisms in biology. Regardless of the organism under study—mammal, amphibian, insect, or worm—the same kinds of protein factors are used to transmit, receive, and interpret developmental signals. Moreover, as is also true for mechanisms governing growth, inappropriate activity of differentiation and developmental mechanisms can contribute to the production of a cancer cell.

TISSUE MAINTENANCE IN ADULT ORGANISMS

Once an organism can be said to be fully formed, how does it sustain the number of differentiated cells in each tissue and organ for the remainder of its life span? Do all of its cells survive and function for its full lifetime? Or do some cells in each tissue retain the potential to generate replacements for others that become superannuated?

In many complex organisms, such as mammals, both situations may be found. Neurons of the central nervous system simply decline in number as some expire with age; there is little or no replacement. In organs like the liver, mature cells retain the capacity to duplicate and thus to replenish those lost by attrition or injury. Most commonly, fully differentiated cells lose their ability to undergo further rounds of cell division; they may then function only for several days or weeks, and upon their death must be replaced through the division of cells that are less fully advanced along their differentiation pathway. This continual loss of mature, differentiated cells requires that developmental processes be recapitulated even in adult organisms, especially those with relatively long life spans.

Replenishment of differentiated cells is generally accomplished by supplying each tissue and organ with a smaller cohort of relatively primitive cells (stem cells) that in some ways resemble cells in a developing embryo. Stem cells in adult tissues possess a dual potential: to differentiate along at least one pathway and to duplicate *without* progression toward a fully differentiated state. Thus a stem-cell division

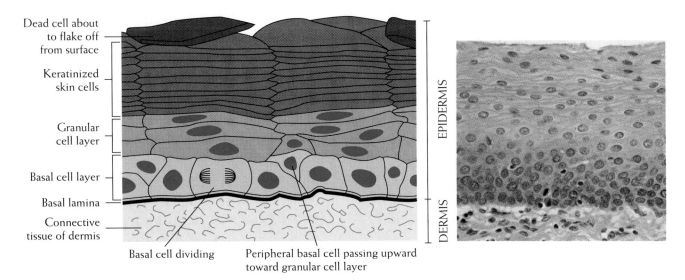

Dead cell about to flake off from surface
Keratinized skin cells
Granular cell layer
Basal cell layer
Basal lamina
Connective tissue of dermis

EPIDERMIS
DERMIS

Basal cell dividing   Peripheral basal cell passing upward toward granular cell layer

A section of human skin seen through the light microscope (right) and depicted schematically (left). Dividing stem cells both renew their own numbers and produce nondividing mature epithelial cells, which rise toward the skin surface, lose their nuclei, and die.

cycle may produce one daughter cell that is identical with the parental cell that it replaces and one daughter cell that assumes the differentiated traits of mature cells in the organ in question. Both replication and differentiation require complex regulation. The organism as a whole must control the frequency with which stem cells undergo rounds of division that maintain or expand their numbers (self-renewal). And it must control the frequency with which the offspring of stem cells proceed toward a fully differentiated, nondividing state.

An understanding of differentiation is fundamental to the study of cancer for several reasons. Cancer cells arising in different organs may resemble normal cells at various stages of differentiation, and this resemblance may allow a forecast of the clinical behavior of the tumor. For example, tumor cells that are more primitive than differentiated may be an unfavorable prognostic sign. Furthermore, it is increasingly apparent that the mechanisms governing differentiation are often disrupted during the conversion of a normal cell to a cancer cell.

Progression along a differentiation pathway, with the acquisition of specialized functions, is often accompanied by a concomitant loss of growth potential, implying some need to balance growth and differentiation. Exploiting this balance may offer novel opportunities for therapies against cancer (see Chapter 8). These and other motives have inspired the close study of differentiation in a variety of adult tissues: skin epithelium (where the stem cells lie under layers of progressively more differentiated epithelial cells); gonads (where the precursors to sperm and eggs must undergo meiosis to reduce the size of their genomes by

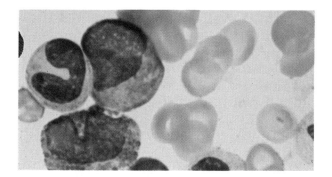

A variety of mature human blood cells arise from a single hematopoietic stem-cell type by division and differentiation.

half); and the bone marrow and spleen, where the hematapoietic (blood-making) stem cells mature to supply the differentiated cells that circulate in the bloodstream.

The hematopoietic system has been an especially attractive one to study: cells are readily obtained; many different cell types are easily recognized by simple microscopic examination; and leukemias and lymphomas, common cancers of the blood system in humans and animals, often produce revealing arrests or distortions of normal hematopoiesis. As a result of intensive work, it is now possible to trace the origins of a large number of mature cell types to several distinct developmental pathways that emanate from a common hematopoietic stem cell. Here is a situation in which the ease of access to the blood and the diversity of blood cells provide an unusual opportunity to observe how the descendants of a single stem cell may end up committed to a range of final differentiated states. One pathway, for example, leads to the production of mature red blood cells (erythrocytes), responsi-

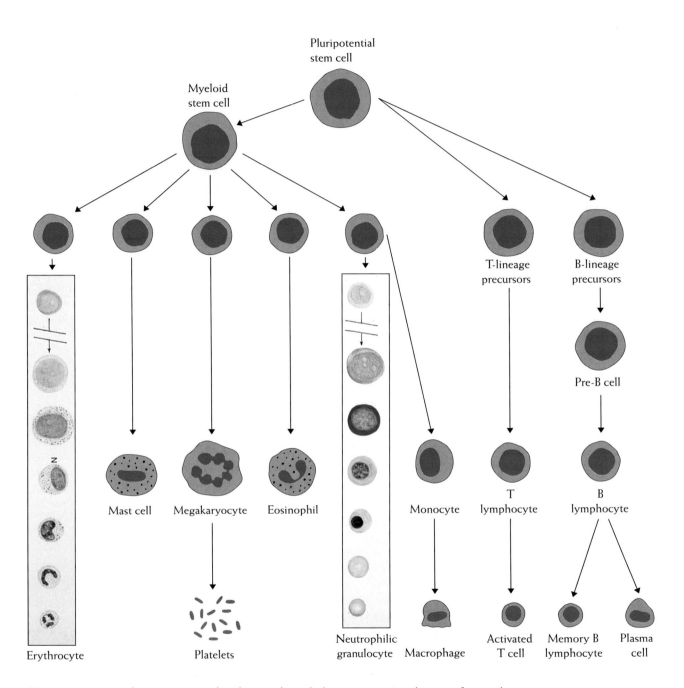

Pluripotential
stem cell

Myeloid
stem cell

T-lineage
precursors

B-lineage
precursors

Pre-B cell

Mast cell   Megakaryocyte   Eosinophil   Monocyte   T
lymphocyte   B
lymphocyte

Erythrocyte   Platelets   Neutrophilic
granulocyte   Macrophage   Activated
T cell   Memory B
lymphocyte   Plasma
cell

Hematopoiesis in vertebrate organisms takes place mostly in the bone marrow. A wide range of particular extracellular protein factors regulate differentiation pathways for developing cells, ensuring that the mature blood-cell types are produced in appropriate proportions.

ble for carrying oxygen—in a complex with the hemoglobin that endows them with color—from the lungs to distant sites in the body. A second pathway yields platelets, which participate in the clotting mechanism. Another produces at least three kinds of cells containing dense granules in their cytoplasm; these cells—named for the staining properties of the granules (neutrophilic, eosinophilic, and basophilic granulocytes)—form part of the organism's defense against bacterial invasion. Progeny of the hematopoietic stem cell on yet another line of descent, the B and T lymphocytes, are responsible for immune defense against foreign agents, attacking invaders directly (T cells) or through the production of antibodies that circulate in the bloodstream (B cells). Finally, hematopoietic stem cells are the precursors of many scavenger cells scattered throughout the body; these cells (such as macrophages) cleanse tissues of unwanted materials like dead cells and bacteria.

This complex differentiation program introduces a new problem into our consideration of stem cells: the offspring of a single hematopoietic stem cell may be directed into any one of these multiple developmental pathways, leading to the production of distinctly different cell types. To maintain appropriate numbers of the many cellular components of the blood, organisms elaborate a large set of extracellular proteins that signal growth and differentiation of cells in the hematopoietic lineage. About 20 secreted proteins have already been identified as such factors for vertebrate blood cells, each tending to influence a specific cell type at a certain stage of its development, prompting a particular differentiation pathway. For example,

erythropoietin (EPO) stimulates growth and differentiation of a precursor to red blood cells; the stem cell factor (SCF) is one of possibly several that sustain the number and competence of stem cells; and colony stimulating factor-1 (CSF-1) is required for the expansion and maturation of macrophages and other cells derived from the macrophage lineage.

Many of these factors are produced by so-called stromal cells—the fibroblasts and other cells lining the bone marrow cavities in which hematopoiesis occurs—rather than by the blood cells themselves. Aberrant production of these factors or derangements of the molecules that recognize them or interpret their signals often occur in cancer cells of the blood-forming organs. This fact reemphasizes the dire consequences of imbalance in differentiation-regulating mechanisms. Cancers that arise in the hematopoietic system are often recognizable by their differentiated characteristics, implying that cancerous change may have begun through an overproduction of cells already committed to one pathway or another during blood formation. Thus, multiple myeloma is due to an expanded population of antibody-producing cells, B-cell lymphomas are composed of immune cells in an early stage of development, and certain leukemias are overgrowths of cells at various points in granulocytic or erythrocytic differentiation.

Having established, in this chapter, how metazoan organisms use their inherited instructions, written in DNA, to develop into complex adults with multiple tissues capable of self-renewal, we now turn to consider in detail the cancers that result from aberrations of normal growth and development.

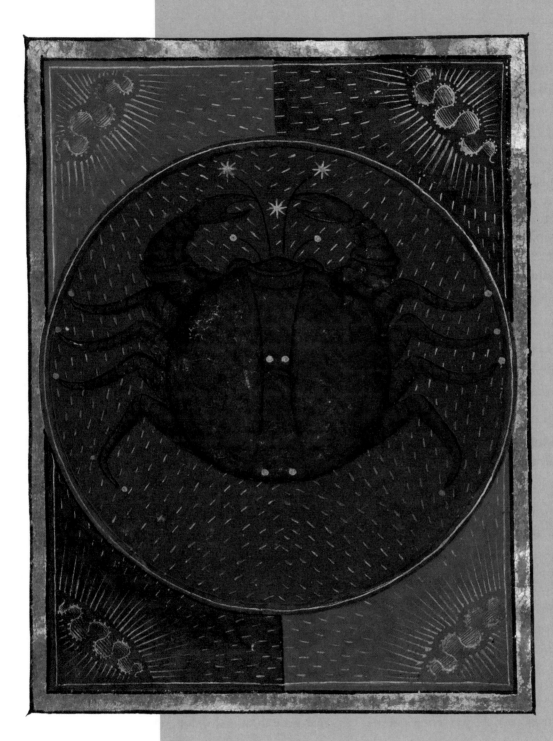

A medieval
manuscript depicts
Cancer, the Crab.

2

THE NATURE OF CANCER

C ancer is a single disease and it is a hundred diseases. The unifying aspect of cancer is uncontrolled growth—the appearance of disorganized tissues that expand without limit, compromising the function of organs and threatening the life of the organism. The hundred faces of cancer come from its appearance in a variety of sites throughout the body. Each cell type, each tissue, may spawn a distinct type of tumor with its own specific growth rate, prognosis, and treatability. To understand cancer, we need to know it close up, at the microscopic level, and ultimately, as we explore it in this book, at the submicroscopic level of deregulated genes and the protein molecules they generate.

TISSUES AND CELLS

Around 400 B.C., Hippocrates likened the long, distended veins radiating from some breast tumors to the limbs of a crab, whence *karkinoma* in Greek and, later, its Latin equivalent *cancer*. But 23 centuries passed before the nature of malignant tumors could be even vaguely comprehended.

Robert Hooke's discovery in 1665 that a slice of cork viewed under the microscope is made of small compartments seeded the idea that living tissues are composed of unit building blocks that he termed cells. By 1837, Hooke's work was generalized to a theory that all living tissues are built up as aggregates of cells.

The modern realization that all living tissues follow a common building plan did little to address the origin of cells in normal and cancerous tissues. As late as the 1840s a number of German pathologists, Rudolf Virchow among them, embraced the idea that cells arise spontaneously from some shapeless extracellular substance, perhaps coagulated from circulating blood. By 1855, however, Virchow had changed his tack, generating an aphorism that was to become a cornerstone of modern biology: "*Omnis cellula a cellula*"—All cells arise from (other) cells. Cells could not arise as spontaneous aggregates of matter, but only through the growth and division of preexisting cells.

In one simple phrase, Virchow struck down a host of theories on the origin of tissues. His dictum forced a simple logic on the developmental plan of complex organisms: all the cells within a mammalian body must arise as direct descendants of a single original cell. Starting with the fertilized egg (zygote), an adult human being of more than 10^{13} cells could be assembled from the products of 45 successive rounds of cell division.

Virchow's logic meant that cancerous tumors, too, must form from cells that descend through a lineage of divisions ultimately traceable back to the zygote. Yet this insight initially provoked more questions than it resolved. How could biologists describe the cell pedigree that begins with a fertilized egg and ends with the mass of cells recognized as a tumor? More specifically, from what kinds of normal cells do tumors descend?

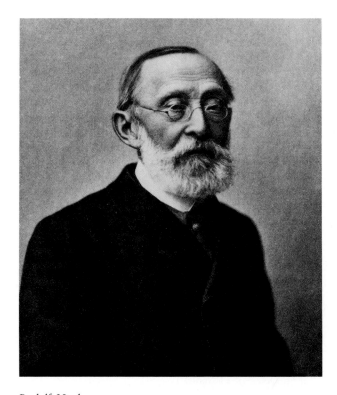

Rudolf Virchow, 1821–1902.

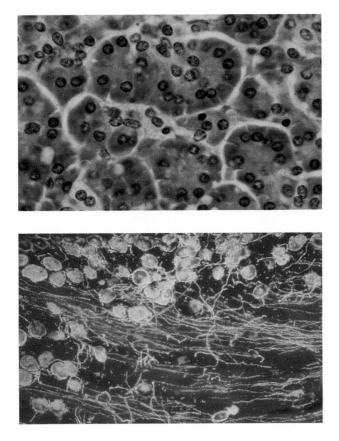

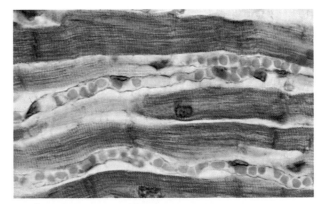

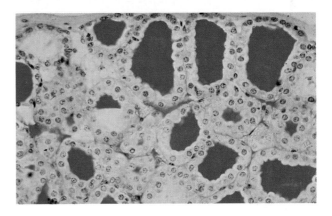

Pathologists like Virchow who studied slices of normal and cancerous tissue led the way in resolving these questions. The trained eye of the pathologist can discern a hundred or more tissue types under the microscope, each defined by a distinct arrangement of cells. One source of this variety is the large number of specialized tissues and organs, but even within a single organ, a variety of normal and abnormal cell types and growth patterns can be discerned.

This diversity of cell types and tissue architectures has two sources. First, a normal organ contains several distinct types of cells that collaborate in its normal functioning. Second, abnormal cell types and growths exist that in one way or another are tied to the process of cancer. To illustrate, we will use the colon as an example, because so much is known about carcinogenesis in this organ. Colon cancer is among the most common types encountered in the West; unlike in other internal organs, moreover, the normal and abnormal states of the colon can be monitored nonsurgically, through colonoscopy.

Carcinogenesis in the Colon

In a normal colon, epithelial cells that line the colon wall continually die and are sloughed off, as occurs in normal skin. To compensate for this loss, cell division occurs in deep pits (crypts) scattered throughout the surface of the epithelium, at the bottom of which primitive, undifferentiated stem cells are continually dividing. Cells recently formed at the bottom of a crypt stop dividing and migrate slowly up the sides toward the surface of the gut epithelium. As they migrate, they develop the ability to absorb nutrients and water and begin to secrete the mucous layer protecting the gut lining. These recently differentiated cells then replace their predecessors.

Both anatomical and morphological observations show that this process may go astray, resulting in the thickened patches of epithelial cells known as polyps or adenomas. The more

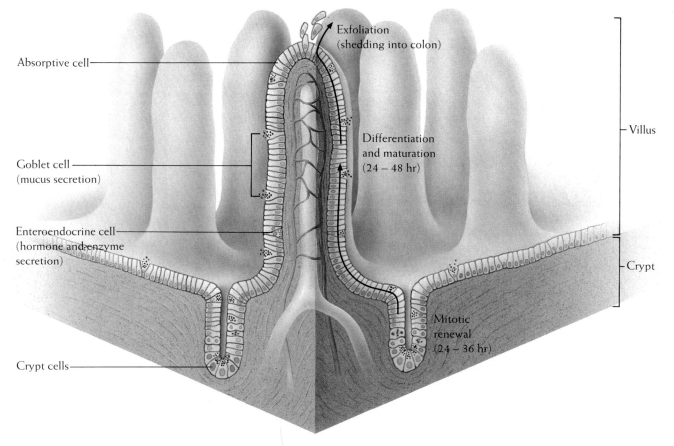

Absorptive cell

Goblet cell
(mucus secretion)

Enteroendocrine cell
(hormone and enzyme
secretion)

Crypt cells

Exfoliation
(shedding into colon)

Differentiation
and maturation
(24 – 48 hr)

Mitotic
renewal
(24 – 36 hr)

Villus

Crypt

Cell division at the bottom of an intestinal crypt continually renews the epithelium of the villus. Surface cells, migrating upward, stop dividing and differentiate to perform specific functions, including the absorption of nutrients and the secretion of mucus, hormones, antibodies, and enzymes. After a day or two, they die and are shed into the cavity of the gut.

undifferentiated and atypical the cells in such polyps, the greater the potential danger of their continued proliferation.

The real cancers—the carcinomas—almost always arise from secretory cells in the epithelium and thus are termed adenocarcinomas. At best, they carry still recognizable glandlike structures that produce mucus; at worst, they are formed from a fully undifferentiated, or anaplastic, jumble of cells.

The most disquieting fact about carcinomas is that they do not respect territorial boundaries. They begin to grow into the underlying muscle layer of the colonic wall and eventually, progressing further, yield small clumps of progeny cells able to start new colonies—so-called metastases—in other organs. These progeny cells travel through blood or lymph

vessels that drain from the colon—or, more rarely, float through the fluid in the abdominal cavity—to lodge at distant sites. The resulting metastatic growths account for 90 percent of patient deaths from colon carcinoma.

Colon cancer is clearly not a single entity. Rather, a variety of abnormal tissues found in the gut may differ minimally or profoundly from its normal lining. For the moment, we must assume that the peculiarities of each of these growths directly reflect abnormalities in the cells that compose it. We defer the intricacies of *how* these cells arise and focus instead on a more elementary question: *Where* do these abnormal cells come from? Do cancer cells descend from cells in adjacent normal tissue, or are they introduced into the body through infection from another individual?

One answer came from attempts to transplant tissues from one human being to another. Such transplants work well between identical twins, occasionally between genetically related individuals, and rarely when the donor and

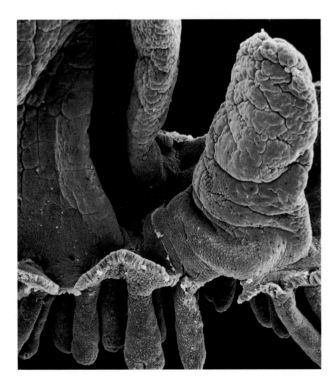

Scanning electron microscope view of a villus in the intestinal epithelium (right) with numerous crypts (below and left). Precancerous change begins with abnormal expansion of cell division from the base (not shown) of a crypt to the top, followed by localized thickening (a polyp) if the dividing, relatively undifferentiated cells spill out to cover the colon surface. Overproliferating (hyperplastic) polyps are benign; cancerlike (neoplastic) adenomas range from small, tubular, secretory polyps through an intermediate tubulovillous stage to large villous polyps. Increase in size correlates with poor cell differentiation and the likelihood of development into cancer.

Metastasis and Prognosis in Colon Cancer

Description of Carcinoma	Percentage of Patients Alive 5 Years after Diagnosis
Limited to mucosal lining of gut	100
Extending down to underlying muscle layer but not penetrating through it; no lymph nodes involved	66
Extending down through the muscle layer; no cancer cells in nearby lymph nodes	53.9
Invading through the muscle wall and beyond, with occasional involved nearby lymph nodes	42.8
Invasion as above with cancer cells in many local nodes	22.4
As above with distant metastatic spread to (in declining order of likelihood) liver, lung, bones, the peritoneal membrane of the abdomen, and the brain	4

Based on the Dukes staging scheme, a clinical estimate.

recipient are unrelated. The barrier to transplantation arises because the recipient's immune system can distinguish between cells of foreign origin and those that have always lived in the host. Once a donor cell is recognized as alien, it is quickly destroyed.

Accordingly, an individual's tissues can be classified or "typed" on the basis of whether they can be grafted into another person's body. Tissues of identical twins are typed as identical: they can be freely exchanged between the twins. Tissue-typing tests reveal that the tumor cells of a cancer patient are always of the same special transplantation type as the cells of normal tissues elsewhere in the patient's body. This fact is a persuasive argument that the cells forming the tumor are indigenous, not invaders from another body. We can conclude that tumors arise from normal tissues. But how does this occur?

THE ORIGINS OF TUMOR CELLS

Two scenarios describe how cancers might derive from normal tissue. According to the first, a large cohort of normal cells within a tissue may be recruited by some unknown agent into becoming cancer cells. The cells seen later in a clinically obvious tumor would be the descendants of this large group of ancestral cells, each of which crossed over the threshold from normality to malignancy during this earlier recruitment. Since the lineal descendants of each individual ancestral cell form a single homogeneous population known as a cell clone, the tumor as a whole—formed as a composite of multiple cell clones—is said to have a polyclonal makeup.

The alternative scheme proposes that all the cells in a tumor are the descendants of a single ancestor that underwent conversion from a normal to a cancerous state. These cells, which may number more than 100 billion in a large tumor, are members of a single lineage and can thus be said to form a monoclonal population.

To choose between these two models using most experimental techniques can be exceed-

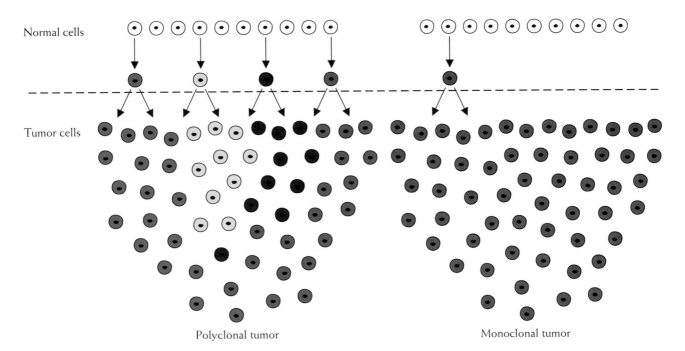

Normal cells

Tumor cells

Polyclonal tumor   Monoclonal tumor

Two schemes by which tumorigenesis could occur. In the first (left), four normal cells independently become transformed and the progeny of each contribute to the tumor mass. In the second (right), a single cell undergoes transformation and becomes the ancestor of all the cells in the tumor. Most—perhaps all—human cancers appear to be monoclonal in origin.

ingly difficult. If a tumor were polyclonal, how could the clones be distinguished from each other? More to the point, how could the cells forming one clone be distinguished from those of another? Occasionally it is possible to tell clonal cells apart when certain cells bear some unique distinguishing mark—a readily recognizable aberration.

Finding such distinguishing marks can be very challenging for a researcher surveying the cells of one type (for example, epithelial) within a normal tissue: they appear, for all practical purposes, identical. Tumor cells, on the other hand, often do acquire distinctive abnormalities seen rarely if ever in normal tissue. The most readily visualized of these markings are random aberrations in the structure of certain chromosomes, which seem to arise spontaneously during the growth of a tumor.

In certain instances, all the cells forming a tumor carry chromosomes having the same, very unusual chromosome rearrangement. This aberration sets these cells apart from their normal counterparts in the tissue and, more importantly, provides an unambiguous indication that these tumor cells all descend from a common ancestor that, through some random accident, suffered this alteration. This represents clear proof that a particular tumor is indeed monoclonal in origin.

MONOCLONAL TUMORS

In fact, virtually all malignant tumors are now thought to be monoclonal in origin. This is often difficult to prove, because most tumor cells lack obvious distinguishing marks like chromosomal aberrations. But there is a clever way to prove the monoclonality of virtually all types of tumors that depends upon a peculiarity of sexual genetics in mammals, including human beings.

Men have one and women two X chromosomes in all their somatic cells. (In males, the maternal X is paired with a paternal Y chromosome.) These X chromosomes determine sex, but they also carry additional genes essential for normal body functions. This creates a quandary. Women have two copies of each X-associated gene (one from each parent), while men have only one, yet the products of these genes will often be needed in equal amounts in male and female tissues. How does nature prevent female cells, with their double copy, from having twice as much of the products of these X-linked genes?

Female mammals solve this problem by silencing one of the two X chromosomes in each of their cells; virtually all the genes on a silenced X chromosome are shut down. While a silenced X chromosome is still present in each female cell, its genes are fully inactive and thus, in effect, absent. Female cells are thereby functionally reduced to the same single-X state seen in male cells.

This X-chromosome inactivation takes place randomly in female embryos very early in development. Some cells and their lineal descendants within a tissue have the maternal X chromosome repressed; others repress the paternal one. If the two X chromosomes carry slightly different information, the two types of cells will be distinguishable from one another, depending upon which of their X chromosomes has been silenced.

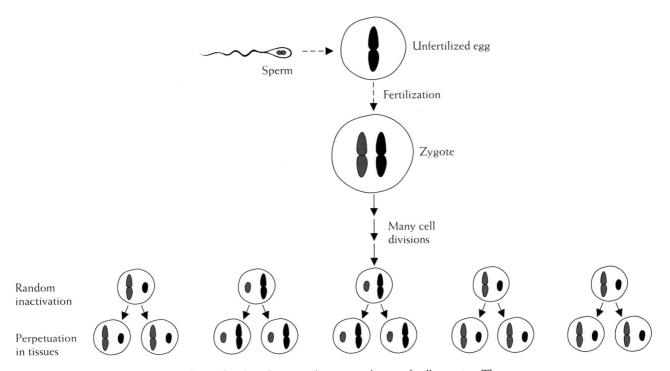

X-chromosome inactivation occurs after a female embryo reaches many dozens of cells in size. The maternal or paternal X chromosome is inactivated at random, but all descendants of each inactivated embryonic cell preserve the pattern of X silencing sustained by their ancestor.

Scientists have found that all the cells within a given tumor invariably have the same X chromosome inactivated. On this basis, they could conclude that all cells in the tumor must descend from a single ancestral cell that had silenced this particular X chromosome. Once again, it was possible to conclude that malignant tumors are monoclonal. (Similar conclusions apply to a variety of benign growths that have been studied.)

The picture emerging from all this is that a single normal cell undergoes conversion into a cancer cell. Its descendants, proliferating over many years, produce a large population of cells, each identical to the others and all faithful replicas of their common ancestor. This cell population in aggregate constitutes a tumor mass that creates the symptoms of cancer.

This simple picture, essentially correct, needs to be refined further. Although all cells within a tumor mass may well share a distinctive mark (the same chromosomal aberration or X-chromosome inactivation), detailed comparison of cells from different sectors of a tumor mass may also show regional differences in appearance. Observations like these force us to consider a more sophisticated model of tumor formation.

As a tumor develops, the initial monoclonal population of cells may become more and

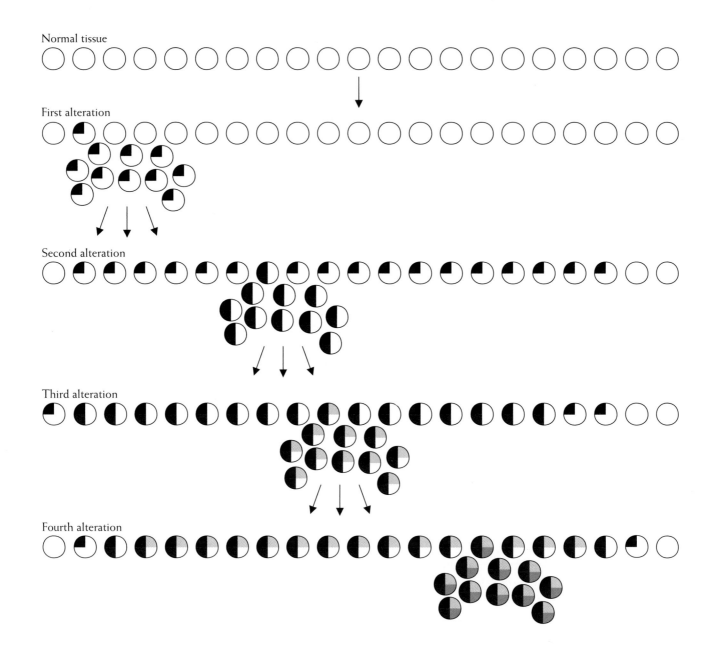

Normal tissue

First alteration

Second alteration

Third alteration

Fourth alteration

Scheme of how a cell clone may sustain successive multiple alterations (mutations) in its genome—in this case, four—that allow it to compete with increasing success against cells that lack the full complement of mutations. Tumor progression is shown to equal a series of clonal expansions analogous to Darwinian evolution in response to natural selection.

more heterogeneous as its descendants diversify by acquiring new, distinctive traits and form distinct subpopulations within the tumor. There is ample time for these diversifications to occur, since human tumors often become apparent only after they have grown to a size of 10 billion to 100 billion cells. Several decades must pass from the initiation of the tumor to its ultimate detection in the clinic. Often cited in this context is the 20- to 25-year lag between the onset of widespread cigarette smoking among women after World War II and the massive increase in female lung cancer detected in the 1970s.

Cancer cells, moreover, have been found to be genetically unstable. While normal cells maintain a fixed, stable complement of chromosomes and displayed traits over dozens of cell generations, tumor cells seem intrinsically erratic, prone to rearrange, duplicate, and delete portions of their chromosomes during cell division and, as a consequence, to display novel, even bizarre, traits in their progeny cells. This plasticity, working over the very long period of tumor development, favors great diversification in different branches of the family tree that radiates from the common initiating ancestor cell. The tumor as a whole is monoclonal in origin, but the initial events that created the common ancestral cell would seem to be only the first in a complicated succession that eventually results in a large number of diverse cells among its descendants.

When novel or distinguishing traits acquired by a cancer cell help it to grow and divide efficiently, these traits will be represented increasingly among the competing cell populations in a tumor. Indeed, the development of a tumor is often likened to the process of evolution. Many of the new traits acquired during the process of tumor development—often termed tumor progression—allow the affected cell to grow more rapidly and thereby to compete more effectively with normal cells and other premalignant cells nearby. This natural selection occurring within the confines of a tissue ultimately creates cells able to dominate their surroundings and proliferate without limit. In practice, of course, tumor cell populations sooner or later exceed the ability of the host to nourish them. Often long before that, tumors will compromise the functioning of a vital organ, leading first to illness and then to death.

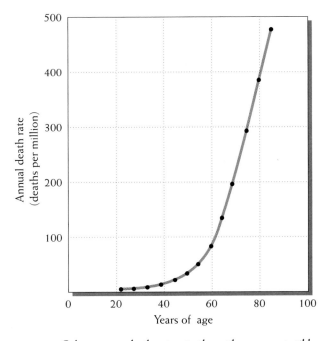

Colon cancer deaths rise steeply with age, compatible with multistep, time-dependent tumor progression.

Why Are There So Many Types of Cancer?

Each of the many cell types within the body provides a potential site for the formation of a tumor, which is then categorized by the tissue from which it arose. Of the four major types, listed below with examples of the tumors they may form, epithelial cells generate more than 90 percent of human cancers. Are they inherently more susceptible to growth deregulation? Certainly their exposed locations put them in direct contact with many carcinogenic agents.

CELL TYPE	TISSUE	DERIVED TUMORS
Epithelial	Breast (milk secretion)	Adenocarcinomas (from
	Liver (bile secretion)	secretory tissue)
	Skin	Squamous carcinomas (from
	Linings of stomach, gut,	protective linings)
	bladder, lung, uterus	
Connective tissue	Cartilage	Chondrosarcomas
	Bone	Osteosarcomas
	Muscle	Rhabdomyosarcomas
	Blood vessel	Angiosarcomas
Blood-forming	Bone marrow; spleen (may	Lymphomas, myelomas,
	spill into circulation)	erythroleukemias, lymphocytic
		and myelogenous leukemias
Nerve	Peripheral nervous system	Neuroblastomas
	(spinal cord ganglia,	
	adrenal cortex)	
	Central nervous system	Gliomas, astrocytomas,
	(notably brain)	medulloblastomas, neuromas,
		schwannomas

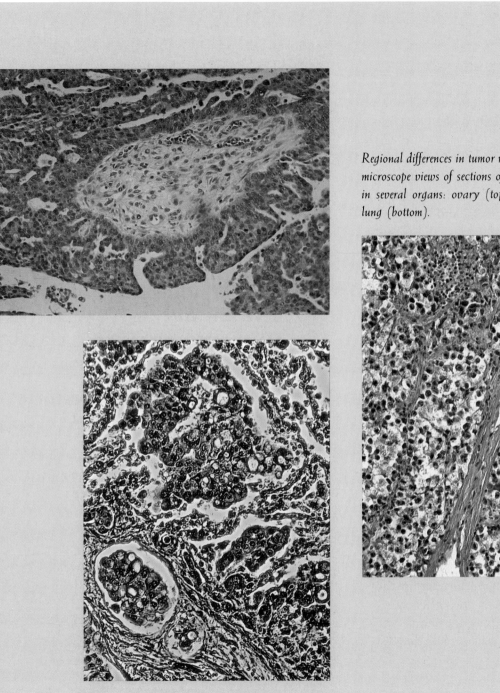

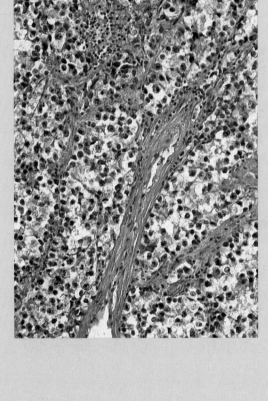

Regional differences in tumor mass are reflected in light microscope views of sections of human cancers arising in several organs: ovary (top), testicle (center), and lung (bottom).

ABNORMALITIES OF CANCER CELLS

This description of tumor development suggests that cancer cells differ from their normal counterparts in a number of attributes, some of which are inextricably linked to the capacity for uncontrolled growth. Much cancer research over the past half century has focused on cataloguing the many differences between normal and tumor cells. Initially, these studies concentrated on individual tumor cells and their appearance in a tissue—their shapes; the form of their nuclei; the arrays they assume within the tumor mass.

Cancer cells often show a profound shift in the relationship between their nuclei and their cytoplasms. In many normal cells, the nucleus is much smaller than its cytoplasm, often only one-fifth as large; in many cancer cells, the nucleus is almost as large as the whole cell, with only a small cytoplasmic rim around it. Analysis often shows increased amounts of DNA per tumor cell, reflecting an abnormal increase in chromosomal number, and the nuclei carrying this DNA may take on a variety of unusual shapes. Significantly, an unusually high percentage of cells in a tumor are undergoing mitosis. Normal tissues, by contrast, usually have a low, even undetectable, percentage of dividing cells.

As we noted earlier when considering the colon, cancer cells often lack the differentiated, specialized traits of their ancestors. Secretory cells often release mucus, but derived adenocarcinomas may have lost this trait. Connective tissue tumors may no longer make collagen as their normal counterparts do. While epithelial cells usually contain large amounts of keratin, the derived squamous carcinomas may no longer accumulate this protein in their cytoplasms.

In sum, cancer cells often lose organ- or tissue-specific traits. The energies of these cells are directed exclusively toward their own proliferation; they no longer focus on helping to build a functional organ or tissue. This loss of differentiated traits often signals the presence of what is termed a high-grade, aggressive tumor, with poor associated prognosis for the patient.

THE ORIGIN OF UNDIFFERENTIATED CELLS

The relatively undifferentiated state of certain tumor cells is reminiscent of the state of embryonic cells prior to their specialization during development. But how do these undifferentiated cells arise? We might consider them as having reverted to a more primitive state of differentiation. In this view, such a cell has evolved backward, shedding many of the attributes and specialized functions that it and its forebears acquired during embryonic development. This process is often called dedifferentiation.

But there is another, equally compelling view of these undifferentiated tumor cells. In most fully developed adult organs, the continued loss of differentiated, functional cells is balanced by the proliferation of stem cells like those growing at the bottom of the colonic crypts. Stem cells are usually relatively undifferentiated in appearance and function. Most fully differentiated cells have lost their ability to divide, but stem cells divide seemingly without limit; some of their offspring take on differentiated traits. In one sense, these stem cells represent small islands of embryonic cells amid a sea of differentiated cells in the adult tissue.

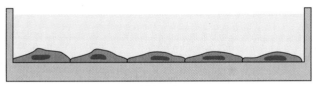

Normal

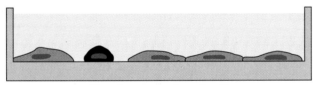

Transformation of single cell

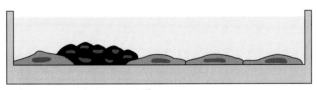

Focus

Side view of cells growing in a petri dish. Lacking the contact inhibition of normal cells, transformed cells proliferate to form a thick focus visible to the naked eye.

Knowing this, one can portray cancer cells in a different light: perhaps they have arisen as a consequence of arrested differentiation. Perhaps such cells have not moved backward from a more to a less differentiated state, but instead act like stem cells whose normal differentiation has been blocked. They may be trapped in a stem-cell-like state, prevented from ever differentiating but with an unlimited ability to divide.

NORMAL AND CANCER CELLS IN CULTURE

Descriptions of cancer cells as they exist within living tissues are unrevealing in one very important respect: they present a static view of the cancer process, a description of the end products of several decades of tumor development. We need a complementary, dynamic view that can come only from looking at the living cancer cell—something that is impossible when that cell is embedded deep within a tumor mass or mounted on a microscope slide.

Considerations like these have prompted cancer biologists to grow living cells outside the body. Such in vitro culture—the term recalls the early use of glass petri dishes—allows tumor cells to be maintained and propagated for extended periods and their vital properties to be studied with great precision. This has yielded an abundance of data that helps explain how cancer cells differ from their normal counterparts.

The differences between contrasting communities formed by normal and cancer cells in culture are most dramatic when viewing fibroblasts (connective tissue cells), which are particularly easy to grow in culture. Most normal tissues are composed of well-ordered layers of cells. Normal fibroblasts attempt to recapitulate this arrangement within the confines of a culture dish, where they usually form layers precisely one cell thick. Such monolayers are not seen when cancer cells are propagated in culture; tumor cells pile up on top of one another. The normal cells clearly have the ability to stop growing when they have covered the surface of the dish, while cancer cells have lost this trait. When normal cells touch each other, they respond by shutting down their growth; such self-control is termed contact inhibition.

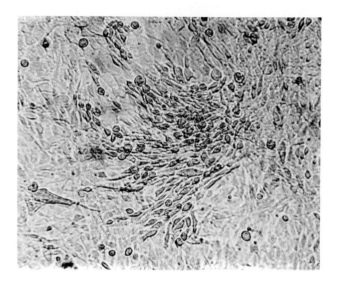

Chick embryo cells in culture that the Rous sarcoma virus has transformed pile up thickly, growing without contact inhibition.

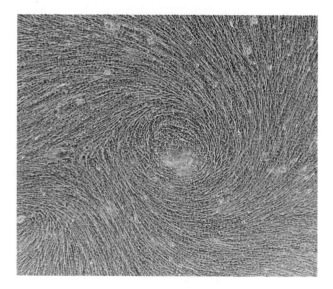

The well-ordered, flat growth pattern of a normal cell monolayer in culture. These are human fibroblasts.

When a tumor cell is seeded in a petri dish, its descendants, lacking contact inhibition, continue to divide without limit, overgrowing the surrounding monolayer of normal cells and creating the multilayered clump of cells known as a focus. Loss of contact inhibition seems to represent the essence of the cancer state—failure of the ability to respond to environmental cues by stopping growth.

But the loss of contact inhibition is only one of many aberrations in growth control. Another, possibly related phenomenon is seen when both normal and malignant cells are seeded into a gelatin or agar matrix, deprived of direct contact with the surface of the culture dish. Normal cells placed in such a suspension will remain alive but will not divide;

tumor cells will usually grow nicely, forming a ball of descendants.

Having gained the ability to grow without direct contact with a solid substrate, these tumor cells are said to be anchorage-independent, in contrast to their normal, anchorage-dependent counterparts. Once again, tumor cells relate to their surroundings in a way dramatically different from that of their normal ancestors.

An equally striking difference comes from examining the composition of the medium that, added to the culture dish, enables these various cells to grow. All mammalian cells, normal or cancerous, require a common set of nutrients, including glucose, vitamins, and

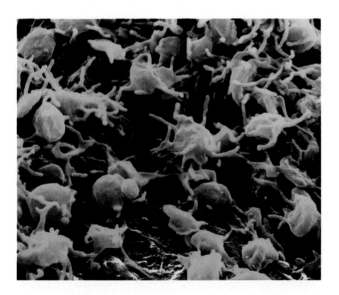

Activated blood platelets on damaged epithelial tissue release a variety of growth-stimulating factors. These serum factors can be used to prompt cells to grow in culture.

amino acids. But these alone usually do not suffice in culture, and calf serum is almost always required to complete the cocktail. Calf serum does not contain nutrients but instead supplies so-called growth factors that stimulate the cells to divide in culture. As we will see in Chapter 6, these serum growth factors mimic similar factors used by cells in normal tissues to stimulate each other's growth. In their absence, cells will be viable, with an active metabolism, but will not proliferate.

Significantly, tumor cells usually display a greatly decreased dependence on serum and its associated growth factors; some types can grow with almost none. This growth-factor autonomy is yet another way that cancer cells relate to their environment profoundly differently. The growth of tumor cells seems to be regulated by some internal program, not by cues from the external environment that are communicated by growth factors.

The internal organization of the individual cancer cell grown in culture is also distinctive. The structure of all cells—their cytoarchitecture—is determined by the network of proteins that assemble to form the cytoskeleton. Very important components of a fibroblast cytoskeleton are intracellular cables composed of assemblies of the protein actin. These actin cables are found in ordered arrays in normal cells; in tumor cells derived from fibroblasts, these cables seem disorganized and in many places are nonexistent.

Near the cell's periphery, the cytoskeleton is connected via protein couplers to receptors on the outside cell surface. These receptors tether the cell to a substrate or to the protein networks that aggregate, forming the extracellular matrix. Such adhesion is often greatly reduced in tumor cells, with the result that cancer cells growing in the culture dish often display quite rounded, distinct borders, seen in the microscope as a shiny, refractive halo. Normal cells, by contrast, are quite spread out and well adhered to the substrate; their flatness is a sign of their normality.

More subtle changes in cell behavior cannot be visualized so readily and must be detected using biochemical techniques. One well-known example is a feature discovered by the German biochemist Otto Warburg in the 1930s. To produce energy, he found, cancer cells frequently metabolize sugars like glucose without concomitant consumption of oxygen. Such anaerobic glycolysis, which results in production of lactic acid, distinguishes many cancer cells from their normal counterparts,

which use oxygen to burn sugars and thereby release carbon dioxide. Warburg argued that anaerobic glycolysis provided an explanation of the malignant state—indeed was a cause of it—but we now believe that it is only one of many secondary consequences of the transition to malignancy.

One final idiosyncrasy of cancer cells merits special attention: they can often proliferate indefinitely in culture. Normal cells seem to be governed by a growth program that limits them to a fixed number of divisions in culture before they become senescent and die. No one fully understands this limited proliferative ability of normal cells and the contrasting growth program of tumor cells. The ability to divide for a seemingly unlimited number of generations, termed cellular immortality, seems to represent an important component of the neoplastic state, allowing a tumor to expand with-

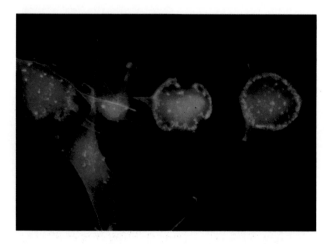

Immunofluorescence (green) displays the actin within mouse fibroblasts. The cells above, transformed by the SV40 large-T oncogene, have become rounded, with cytoskeletons disorganized.

The cells below have reverted from a transformed state back to normal appearance and show well-organized cytoskeletons, although they still carry SV40 large-T oncoprotein (orange) in their nuclei.

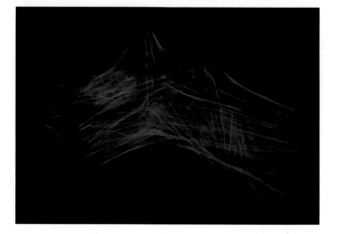

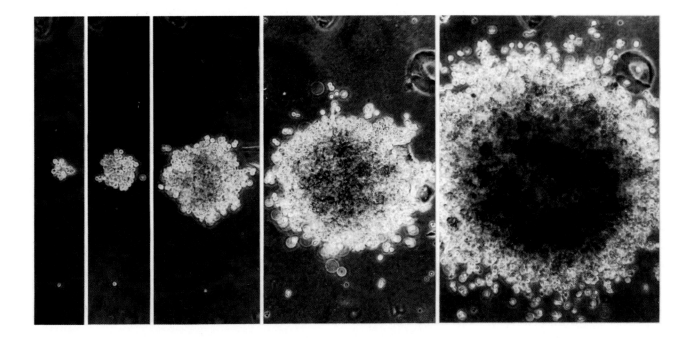

Normal cells cannot grow unless they adhere to a solid substrate. These transformed cells, expanding into a globular colony within a semiliquid agar suspension, show anchorage-independent growth.

out the constraints imposed by the normal cellular growth program.

In describing these attributes of a typical cancer cell, we seem to ignore the fact that cancer is a collection of a hundred distinct diseases, each involving a different type of malignant cell. It is, however, a thesis of modern cancer research, hardly proved but nonetheless repeated often throughout this book, that certain common mechanisms underlie the formation of all cancers. This unifying principle means that lessons learned from studying one type of cancer cell are often directly transferable to understanding many others.

This view relies upon the fact, established in Chapter 1, that the biology of cell types throughout the body is similar, independent of location or specialized function—a similarity that extends to the heart of the cell and the molecular mechanisms governing cell growth, which seem to be disrupted in very similar ways in tumors that are otherwise very different from one another. Evidence continues to confirm that the cellular machinery regulating cell growth evolved more than a billion years ago, long before the development of many specialized cell types, and has been preserved and adapted for use by various, otherwise very distinctive types of cells. In the next chapter, we begin to trace how the cell's growth-regulating mechanisms are disrupted: How does cancer begin?

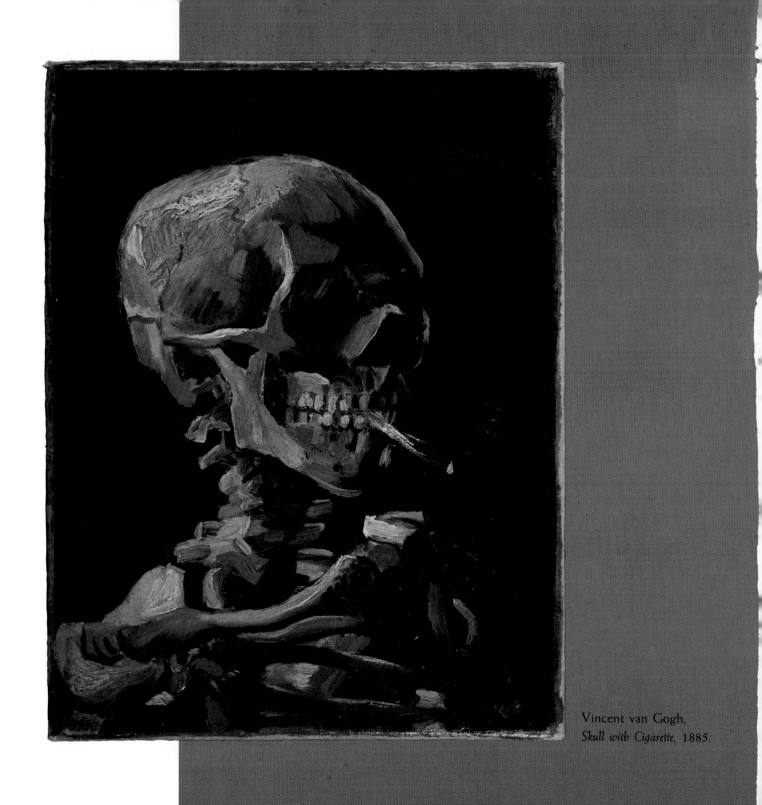

Vincent van Gogh,
Skull with Cigarette, 1885.

CLUES TO THE ORIGIN OF CANCER

3

In 1775 Percivall Pott, a London physician, described an extraordinarily high incidence of scrotal cancer among men who had worked as chimney sweeps during boyhood. In the mid-nineteenth century, pitchblende miners in eastern Germany were observed to die at extremely high rates from lung cancer. By the latter part of the century, snuff and cigar smoking were thought by some medical practitioners to be closely linked to the development of oral cancers.

As these anecdotal reports of association between certain cancers and specific occupations became more numerous, many people began to perceive cancer as arising from sources outside the body; this idea moved beyond earlier dogmas that cancer was exclusively a breakdown of the body's internal machinery, uninfluenced by the outside world. This new way of thinking was important in a second respect: it suggested that cancer could be tied to specific, even identifiable, causes. Thirty years after Percivall Pott's report, a physician noted that chimney sweeps in continental Europe had scrotal cancer rates only half those of their English counterparts and argued that the custom of taking frequent baths, much more prevalent on the Continent, might wash away the offending agent, ostensibly the creosote tars from flues.

CAN EXTERNAL AGENTS CAUSE CANCER?

Once external agents were perceived to provoke cancer, a wide variety of sources came under scrutiny. Coal tar, mine dust, and tobacco were not the only possible culprits. The discoveries of Louis Pasteur and Robert Koch at the end of the nineteenth century that bacteria cause tuberculosis, cholera, typhus, and diphtheria persuaded many physicians that cancer, too, was an infectious disease and that a cancer bacillus would soon be isolated. Indeed, the first American cancer hospitals were founded out of a widely perceived need to quarantine cancer patients.

A rival view held that tumors arise from chronic irritation of tissues. The frequent oral and throat cancers of pipe and cigar smokers reinforced this theory; the searing heat of tobacco smoke was considered a potent irritant. But the nature or source of irritation was rarely agreed upon. The oral cancer that killed U.S. President Ulysses S. Grant was attributed by one expert not to his lifelong penchant for large cigars, but to the constant irritation provoked by the rough surface of a broken tooth.

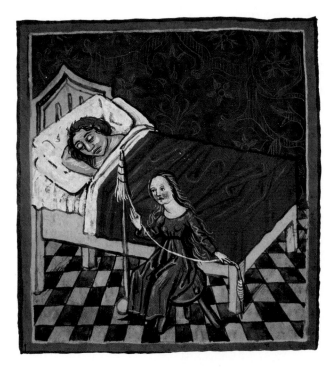

In the third century A.D., *the Greco-Roman physician Galen proposed understanding cancer as an imbalance among the body's four vital fluids, or "humors"— blood, phlegm, yellow bile, and black bile. Tumors arose, he argued, when an excess of black bile (literally,* melancholy) *spread throughout the body: a theory that influenced medical thinking into modern times by characterizing cancer as systemic—a pathology of the body as a whole, rather than a localized breakdown of normal order in a tissue—and linking tumor development to depression.*

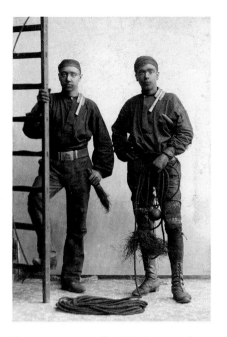

Chimney sweeps suffered high rates of scrotal cancer.

The theory that irritation represents an essential precursor to cancer received a strong boost following the 1895 discovery of X rays by Wilhelm Röntgen and their use almost immediately thereafter in diagnosis and therapy. It soon became clear that direct exposure to X-ray beams would often lead within hours to localized reddening and blistering. By 1902, chronic exposure of the hand of a technician who built and tested X-ray tubes had led to a localized skin cancer. Within a decade, dozens of radiologists and X-ray experimentalists developed a variety of cancers. Like heat, radiation was perceived to induce localized tissue irritation, which led in turn to the appearance of cancer.

Still another theory came from the work of Charles Darwin, who proposed that evolution is driven by the competition among those who inherit more or less favorable traits from their ancestors. Darwin's ideas were further refined by the 1905 revival of Gregor Mendel's theory of genetics. For the first time, heredity and the inheritance of traits from parents were formulated in simple, ostensibly scientific terms, and by the first decade of this century, a range of ills including alcoholism, drug addiction, mental retardation, vagrancy, and even criminality were categorized as inherited diseases, easily traced through family pedigrees. Cancer, too, was seen as hereditary, and the close relatives of a cancer patient often kept the condition secret, lest the family taint be revealed.

Cancer was increasingly recognized, moreover, as a disease of civilization and luxury, striking down the rich and self-indulgent but sparing those who followed the simple life. By 1907, an early epidemiological study noted much higher rates of cancer among the meat-eating Germans, Irish, and Scandinavians of

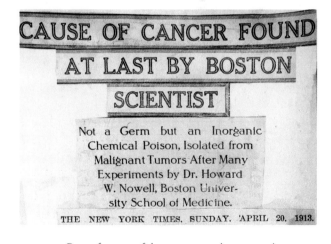

One of many false starts in the twentieth-century search for the origins of cancer.

The view that life style, defined broadly, affects cancer rates can be traced back at least to 1700, when Bernardino Ramazzini in Italy noticed an unusually high rate of breast cancer among nuns and speculated that it related to their celibacy and childlessness. In his words, "You seldom find a convent that does not harbor this accursed pest within its walls." An 1844 report in Verona followed up this observation by compiling uterine and breast cancer rates from the city's death registry for the years 1760 to 1839. The results suggest that married women were more than twice as likely to die of uterine cancer than of breast tumors, while nuns were 9 times more likely to die of breast cancer than of uterine cancer—for nuns, a relative risk of breast cancer 22 times higher.

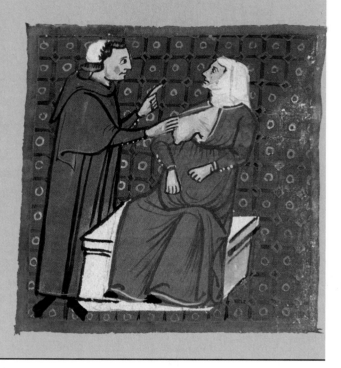

Physicians observed breast cancer at extraordinarily high rates among nuns, in whom cervical cancer almost never was seen.

Chicago than among the city's pasta-eating Italians and rice-eating Chinese. Life style, notably diet, seemed to be an important determinant of risk.

Each early theory of cancer's origin was based upon fragmentary scientific evidence, yet the key observations underlying them ultimately made crucial contributions to our current views and research methods. By correlating disease incidence with epidemiological variables including geography, ethnic origin, diet, habits, life style, occupation, sex, and age, scientists eventually gained unexpected insights into the causation of cancer.

DOES CANCER INCIDENCE VARY?

Perhaps the most important of these insights was the discovery that cancer is a disease showing dramatically differing frequencies in different parts of the globe. Colon cancer is 10 times less common in Nigeria than in Connecticut. Liver cancer, on the other hand, appears 70 times more frequently in Mozambique than in Norway. Stomach cancer rates in Japan are as much as 25 times higher than in Uganda.

Differences in apparent disease incidence might be caused by a number of factors. Indeed, the science of epidemiology works to

Variation in Incidence of Common Cancers

Type of Cancer	Region of Highest Incidence	Risk up to Age 75 (Percent)	Range of Variation[a]	Region of Lowest Incidence
		Men		
Skin	Queensland	Over 20	Over 200	Bombay
Esophagus	Northeast Iran	20	300	Nigeria
Lung	Great Britain	11	35	Nigeria
Stomach	Japan	11	25	Uganda
Liver	Mozambique	8	70	Norway
Prostate	United States (blacks)	7	30	Japan
Colon	Connecticut	3	10	Nigeria
Mouth	India	Over 2	Over 25	Denmark
Rectum	Denmark	2	20	Nigeria
Bladder	Connecticut	2	4	Japan
Nasopharynx	Singapore (Chinese)	2	2	Great Britain
		Women		
Cervix	Colombia	10	15	Israel (Jews)
Breast	Connecticut	7	15	Uganda
Uterus	California	3	30	Japan
Ovary	Denmark	2	6	Japan

[a]The highest incidence observed divided by the lowest incidence observed.

Estimated Importance of Factors Causing Cancer, United States	
Factor	**Percentage of All Cancer Deaths**
Tobacco	30
Alcohol	3
Diet	35
Food additives	Less than 1
Sexual and reproductive behavior	7
Occupation	4
Pollution	2
Industrial products	Less than 1
Medicines and medical procedures	1
Geophysical factors	3
Infection	10 ?
Unknown	?

eliminate as many extraneous, irrelevant factors as possible from consideration. A well-structured epidemiological study would compare, for example, only the disease rate for males in one country with that of males in another, to exclude the sex-linked influence of hormones on disease development. Communities and societies have varying proportions of young and old people; this could skew comparisons because cancer is much more common at later stages of life. To cancel this age effect, cancer rates have come to be calculated in terms of "age-adjusted incidence": What is the risk, for example, of a 40-year-old man in Australia contracting liver cancer compared to that of a 40-year-old man in Bombay?

One other variable still could not be ruled out by such statistics: genetics. Country-by-country variabilities in tumor incidence might be attributable simply to the greatly differing genetic susceptibilities of their inhabitants. But in this case epidemiologists could make use of migrating populations who shifted their homes but, by necessity, carried their genetic baggage with them wherever they went. Japanese-Americans and African-Americans, for example, show cancer rates similar to those of the U.S. population overall and very different from those of genetically close populations in the countries of their ancestry. This showed with clarity that the enormous variability in cancer incidence from country to country derives in large part from environmental differences, rather than from inborn susceptibility. Here the term "environmental" is used to encompass all aspects of an individual's life experience, including the air that is breathed, the water that is drunk, the food that is eaten, and all other aspects of life style and occupation.

By making country-to-country comparisons, epidemiologists could conclude that 70 to 90 percent of American cancer is environmentally caused. For example, if a Central American environment creates a 20-fold lower breast cancer risk than obtains in the United States or Canada, then 95 percent of North American breast cancer can be assumed to have a strong environmental cause that is absent farther

A Cancer Epidemic?

In the eyes of many, statistics suggest an alarming increase of cancer in the general population—a virtual cancer epidemic traceable to modern life style, notably environmental pollution. But careful scrutiny gives a very different picture. The number of new cancer cases every year indeed goes up, in large part because our population is aging: cancer is much more prevalent in old people. Even when adjusted for age, the numbers appear ominous until they are analyzed by tumor type.

Lung cancer deaths are skyrocketing, having increased more than tenfold since 1930 (male/female age-adjusted cases per 100,000 population in 1930 and 1990). More than 90 percent of these cases are related to tobacco smoke. Once the smoking-related tumors are subtracted, however, incidence and death rates for the great majority of other cancers have remained level or declined (leukemia is an exception). Stomach cancer is down by a factor of five to six, apparently because of modern ways of storing and preserving food. Breast cancer mortality rates have been steady, although the rate of new cases detected has gone up, presumably because increased screening detects minute growths that in former years would have remained undetected without threatening life.

Taken together, the data suggest—perhaps unexpectedly—a relatively minor role in human carcinogenesis for the environmental pollutants that have increased substantially over the past half-century.

---

south. By extension, this fraction of cancers could be prevented if the environmental source of breast cancer were determined and eliminated from North America.

Unlike the majority of human cancers, approximately 10 percent—many are cancers of childhood—seem inescapable for all human populations. An unalterable risk of living, they may reflect the multitude of imperfections that our highly evolved bodies still carry.

What, then, are the external influences that incite the great majority of cancers? Their identities could sometimes be revealed by thorough epidemiological studies. Tobacco use comes most rapidly to mind. Its close link to cancer of the mouth, throat, and lung is only one of many such associations uncovered over the past quarter century.

Perhaps the most important impact of such findings was to strengthen the idea that individual tumors can often be traced back to specific, definable first causes. In this sense, cancer no longer had to be viewed as some generalized breakdown of good health caused by a dissolute life style. Simple, discrete causal mechanisms could now be entertained for many common types of human malignant tumors.

Is Cancer Infectious?

While most scientific studies focused increasingly on chemical and physical agents as possible causes of cancer, the infectious theory of human malignancy also witnessed a brief renaissance. This line of work received a scientifically sound, although at the time not widely acclaimed, boost with Peyton Rous's 1910 experiments showing that defined, submicroscopic, filterable agents (that is, viruses) isolated from a chicken sarcoma could induce new sarcomas in healthy chickens.

Despite Rous's discovery of the infectious—specifically viral—nature of the chicken sarcomas, the notion that human cancer is provoked by infectious agents, bacterial or viral, fell into disrepute. Attempts to show that bacteria cause cancer failed, and at the same time it became obvious that the vast majority of human cancers are not contagious. Rous and his work languished in obscurity for half a century before, in 1966, they were recognized with a much-deserved Nobel Prize. By then,

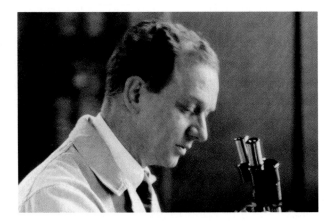

Francis Peyton Rous, 1879–1970.

the infectious theory of cancer had been revived after long neglect. New discoveries showed that viruses besides the "Rous sarcoma virus" could induce cancers in animals. By 1965, polyoma (a mouse virus) and the related simian virus 40 (SV40) had been found to induce a variety of tumors when injected into laboratory rodents, notably mice and hamsters.

Such experiments, profoundly important for all modern thinking about cancer's origins, showed that a tumor could be traced back simply and clearly to a single inciting cause, in this case a particle as small as a virus. Yet they left the important question of mechanisms unanswered: How does a virus trigger a tumor within the complex community of cells that make up a tissue?

Transformation of Cells in Culture

A natural step in answering this question was to study the interaction of cancer-causing viruses with cells growing in culture. Here was the logic driving the work. Since tumors are aggregates of cells, and if the cells in a tumor all descend from a common, aberrant ancestral cell, then the problem of virus-induced cancers should be reducible ultimately to the question of how a virus particle can force a single cell to grow abnormally. Accordingly, the mysterious process triggering cancer in a complex living tissue might be recapitulated in culture and observed through each of its steps.

This strategy succeeded brilliantly. By 1970, investigators had introduced SV40, polyoma, or Rous sarcoma viruses into cultures of

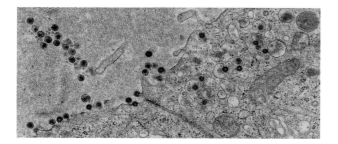

A transmission electron micrograph of an infected cell releasing particles of mouse mammary tumor virus (dark circles) from its plasma membrane (note cell nucleus at bottom).

rodent or chicken cells and observed the resulting foci of altered cells. These clumps showed aberrant shape and growth properties in the petri dish; when they were removed and introduced into animals, they grew into tumors.

This ability to convert normal cells into tumor cells in the culture dish demystified the cancer process. It meant that tumors could be traced back to individual cells that had undergone specific alterations—in this case, infection by one or another "tumor virus." Equally important, these successes meant that the process of transformation, by which a normal cell becomes a tumor cell, could be studied directly. The inception of cancer was no longer inaccessible, hidden within the complex tissues of a living animal.

Most viruses, as we noted in Chapter 1, kill the cells they infect. Yet in the case of these tumor viruses, cells not only survive the initial onslaught of infection but proceed to grow with abnormal vigor—a trait passed on subsequently to all their lineal descendant cells, which might then aggregate to form a tumor mass. How could such viruses permanently mark a cell and all the cell's progeny with the signs of cancer?

THE IMPACT OF THE VIRAL GENOME

By 1960, research on viruses had shown repeatedly that viruses are, in the simplest terms, packets of genes that move from one cell to another. Virus particles are nucleic acid cores (RNA in the case of Rous sarcoma virus; DNA in the case of SV40 and polyoma viruses) carried in a protective coating of proteins and often lipids (fats). The number of distinct genes carried by a single virus particle is small—in the case of these tumor viruses, only three to five—yet is sufficient to induce transformation of a cell in culture.

Two strategies were proposed by which the three to five viral genes might redirect the metabolism of the infected cell's own complement of 50,000 or more genes, transforming it into a cancer cell. In the first, the virus enters the cell, the introduced viral genes irreversibly alter the cell, and then the virus and its genes leave the cell. This "hit and run" transformation requires the virus only to initiate the transformation, not to maintain the transformed state in the initial cell and its descendants. In the other viral transformation strategy, not only do the viral genes initiate transformation, but the continued presence of the viral genome is also required in all descendant cells that continue to show cancerous growth traits.

In fact, this second mechanism was found to be the one used by all tumor viruses. The evidence came from repeated observations that copies of viral genomes could be found in all the cells forming a virus-induced tumor. This meant that the ensemble of viral genes was inserted into the initially infected cell; as the cell proliferated, copies of the viral genome were replicated and distributed to all descendant cells. Any descendants that through some happenstance did not inherit a copy of the viral genome returned to normal growth. Cell transformation, then, might be understood in terms of a small number of viral genes residing inside the cancer cell that issue a continuous stream of instructions forcing the cell to grow malignantly.

The viral model of human cancer pathogenesis focused on the so-called retroviruses. These "reverse" viruses, including the Rous sarcoma virus, carry their genetic information in the form of RNA molecules that they copy into DNA upon infecting a cell. In addition to their ability to pass from cell to cell, transforming each, some retroviruses can enter cells and hide within them in a latent state.

These latent infections are best understood in terms of the unusual molecular biology of the retrovirus growth cycle. Upon entering a cell, the retrovirus particle copies its genomic RNA into double-stranded DNA molecules by means of reverse transcription. The resulting DNA is then inserted into a site in the host-cell chromosomal DNA. This process, termed integration, results in a viral DNA genome—a provirus—that becomes established in the host-cell chromosome and functions like other cellular genes arrayed along the chromosomal DNA.

From the moment of its integration, the chromosome-associated provirus may be expressed, issuing instructions (in the form of messenger RNA molecules) that result in cell transformation and the production of progeny virus particles. As an uncommon alternative, the provirus may remain intact and stably integrated, but latent. Messenger RNA copies will not be issued by the provirus genes, so no effects will be felt from its presence in the cell. Days, weeks, or years later, the expression of a latent provirus may be stimulated by some signal impinging on the cell. The provirus will begin to produce messenger RNA, and a cell that had lacked evidence of viral infection may suddenly release copious virus particles.

Retroviral infection has two further aspects, defined by the type of cell infected. Recall that the germ cells in ovary or testes can, as egg or sperm, contribute to a new embryo, passing genes on to an organism in the next generation. Cells elsewhere in the body are somatic cells, which may proliferate to form a variety of normal tissues but have no opportunity to pass on their genetic information.

Retroviruses infecting somatic cells, then, may establish proviruses that persist in that cell and its descendants within a particular tissue. But an infected germ cell may, via sperm or egg, pass its acquired provirus on to the next generation; in this way, a provirus passed through the germ line may be transmitted like an inherited gene. Such an endogenous provirus can actually become part of the genetic endowment of a species, no less than the other tens of thousands of genes that constitute its genome and define its uniqueness.

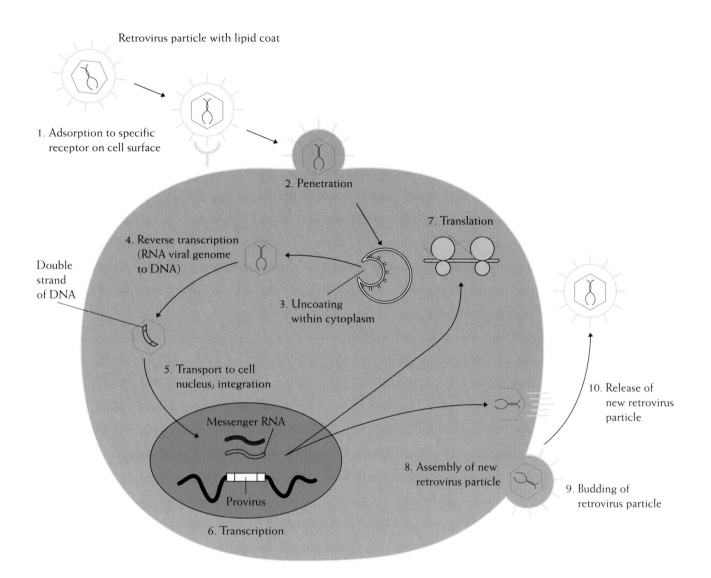

Retrovirus particle with lipid coat

1. Adsorption to specific
   receptor on cell surface

2. Penetration

4. Reverse transcription
   (RNA viral genome
   to DNA)

Double
strand
of DNA

7. Translation

3. Uncoating
   within cytoplasm

5. Transport to cell
   nucleus; integration

Messenger RNA

Provirus

6. Transcription

8. Assembly of new
   retrovirus particle

9. Budding of
   retrovirus particle

10. Release of
    new retrovirus
    particle

The retrovirus life cycle occurs only within a cell. Once the particle core, carrying the viral RNA, is within the cytoplasm, the viral enzyme reverse transcriptase makes a double-stranded DNA copy of the viral RNA genome. This DNA, still in its core, moves to the nucleus and is integrated into the host-cell chromosome as a provirus. Transcription is initiated on the proviral DNA, yielding RNA copies of the viral genome. Some of these RNA molecules move to the cytoplasm where, as messenger RNA, they are translated on cellular ribosomes to synthesize viral proteins. Other viral RNA molecules associate with these proteins, forming a new progeny virus particle, which buds from the plasma membrane.

THE ENDOGENOUS PROVIRUS MODEL

Might the properties of endogenous proviruses make them attractive candidates for the agents that trigger human cancer? Consider one scheme that gained popularity in the late 1960s. Latent endogenous proviruses might become established in the germ line of a species like our own. Exogenous agents such as cancer-causing chemicals enter a cell in one or another tissue of a member of this species, where they may activate a latent endogenous provirus and cause it to be expressed. As a consequence, the cell will begin to produce retrovirus particles and may even be transformed: tumor formation will be initiated. Several chemicals known to be carcinogenic have indeed been found, when applied to mouse or chicken cells, to activate endogenous proviruses, causing these ostensibly uninfected cells to release virus particles.

This endogenous provirus model could also be used to explain heritable human cancers. A number of human tumors seem to occur in familial clusters; the most familiar of these is breast cancer. In these cases, specific genes that confer susceptibility to a specific kind of cancer seem to be passed from generation to generation. Perhaps endogenous proviruses be-

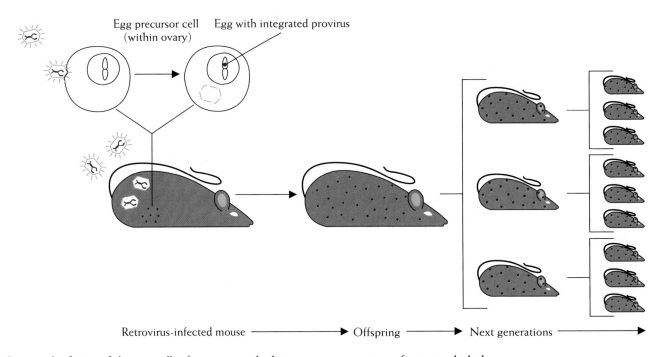

Egg precursor cell (within ovary) Egg with integrated provirus

Retrovirus-infected mouse ⟶ Offspring ⟶ Next generations ⟶

Retroviral infection of the germ cells of a mouse can lead to successive generations of mice in which the acquired provirus is permanently integrated into the mouse DNA genome of every cell.

come established in a family's germ line, thereafter conferring special susceptibility to carcinogenesis in one organ or another.

As it turned out, we humans do carry endogenous proviruses in our germ line, but unlike the proviruses of chickens or mice, they cannot produce infectious virus particles under any condition. Moreover, none of the common cancers, at least those seen in the West, showed clear retrovirus associations, and (with the exception of one cancer—adult T-cell leukemia) extensive attempts to detect retrovirus particles in human tumors failed. The model was abandoned.

Two important legacies remained. Human immunodeficiency virus (HIV), the retrovirus that causes AIDS, was rapidly identified and characterized in the early 1980s, in large part on the basis of knowledge gained from this cancer work in the preceding decade. And many of the genes uncovered in the course of retrovirus research were later found, quite unexpectedly, to play critical roles in human cancer biology. We will return to this subject in Chapter 4.

THE VIROGENE—
ONCOGENE HYPOTHESIS

A version of the endogenous retrovirus model first proposed by Robert Huebner and George Todaro came to be called the virogene–oncogene hypothesis, and it led by a circuitous path to our current insights into cancer's molecular origins. It stated that fragments of endogenous retrovirus genomes lay scattered here and there throughout the mammalian genome as residues of ancient germline infections by retroviruses. Although these fragmented viral genes could not induce the release of retrovirus particles, they might indeed be able to transform the cell, once activated by specific stimuli like those known to turn on latent proviruses. The cancer-causing viral gene fragments were termed oncogenes.

By the end of the 1970s, this virogene–oncogene hypothesis also fell into disrepute, in large part because its detailed predictions could not be sustained by direct molecular analysis. But it hinted at an important idea that eventually found solid confirmation: the normal human genome contains a number of genes that have the ability to direct malignant cell growth.

As for the infectious models of human cancer, careful epidemiologic sleuthing saved some of them in the end. It is now clear that at least four human viruses are inciting factors or cofactors in the formation of specific cancers. Epstein-Barr virus is an agent of Burkitt's lymphoma (sub-Saharan Africa) and nasopharyngeal carcinoma (Southeast Asia); hepatitis B virus is closely associated with liver cancer (worldwide, especially Southeast Asia and Africa); human papilloma viruses contribute to cervical carcinoma (worldwide); and human T-cell leukemia virus, a retrovirus, is a factor in adult T-cell leukemia (Caribbean; southern Japan). But by the late 1970s, it became clear that viruses could not be invoked as prime agents or even intermediaries in provoking the great majority (95 percent) of cancers in Europe and North America. The answers lay elsewhere.

A Viral Link in Liver Cancer

D espite the widely held conviction that viruses are not important causal factors in human cancers, R. Palmer Beasley of Seattle initiated a study of hepatocellular carcinoma (liver cancer) in Taiwan in 1975. Attempting to correlate the incidence of chronic hepatitis B virus (HBV) infection with subsequent death from liver cancer, he enrolled 22,707 men in his study, 3454 of whom were positive for the HBV surface antigen—a sign of chronic viral infection—and 19,253 negative. (Beasley studied male government bureaucrats because liver cancer was three to four times more common in men and a government insurance program monitored their health even after retirement.) By 1986, he had accumulated 202,000 man-years of monitored population data. Of the 161 cases of liver cancer that had developed in these men, 152 were in the HBV-positive population. Virtually all (94 percent) of the cancers arose in the minority of men (15.2 percent) who were HBV positive, demonstrating their risk as 98.4 times higher than those having no apparent infection. The role of chronic HBV infection (and its attendant liver damage) in triggering liver cancer was proved.

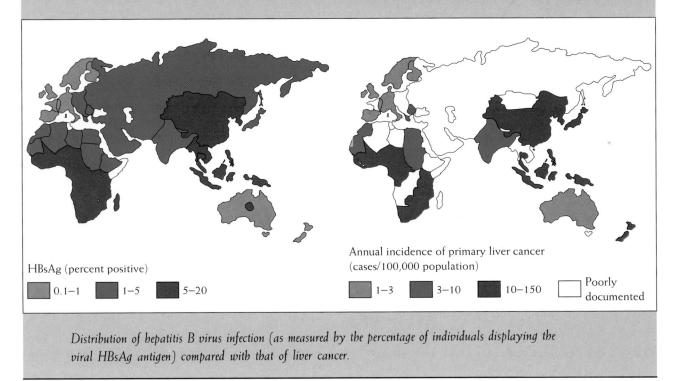

HBsAg (percent positive)

■ 0.1–1   ■ 1–5   ■ 5–20

Annual incidence of primary liver cancer (cases/100,000 population)

■ 1–3   ■ 3–10   ■ 10–150   □ Poorly documented

Distribution of hepatitis B virus infection (as measured by the percentage of individuals displaying the viral HBsAg antigen) compared with that of liver cancer.

X Rays and the Generation of Tumors

The idea that cellular genes play a central role in cancer formation did not flow entirely from work on tumor viruses. A second line of inquiry reached this conclusion using totally different methods, logic, and data. We trace the origins of this model to the turn of the century, before Peyton Rous's work, and to the observation that repeated X-ray exposure correlated with subsequent cancer onset. Numerous anecdotes connecting radiation exposure and cancer continued to accumulate in the following decades, but the various tumors induced by radiation, including skin cancers, leukemias, and bone cancers, were not easily explained by mechanisms of localized irritation; something more subtle seemed to be going on, since tumors sometimes appeared even when no gross irritation was apparent at the irradiated site.

One clue came from the work of Herman Muller at Columbia University, who noted in 1927 that X-irradiation of *Drosophila* fruit flies often resulted in mutant offspring. Such radiation became a useful tool for creating genetic variants, but this work also established that X rays may affect cells (and, by extension, whole organisms) through their ability to damage and thereby mutate genes.

These observations led to the speculation that the two known biological effects of X rays—cancer induction and genetic mutation—might be directly connected. The line of thinking went as follows (surely involving logical leaps and tenuous assumptions). X rays induce mutations in the germ cells of flies, re-

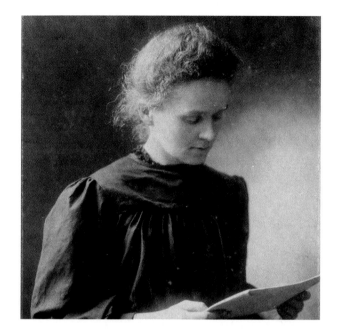

Marie Curie (1867–1934), the first individual to receive the Nobel Prize twice, identified carcinogenic elements in pitchblende.

sulting in offspring that have acquired mutant genes. Radiation should, therefore, be viewed as a mutagenic agent capable of damaging the genetic material inside cells. While the chemical nature of this genetic material was obscure in the 1930s and 1940s, it seemed that similar material, comparably sensitive to X rays, resides in all animal cells, including the normal cells throughout our bodies that are susceptible to radiation carcinogenesis. Accordingly, the cells of radiation-induced tumors might carry mutant genes—genes directly altered by X rays. Some researchers further surmised that chemical carcinogens might create cancer through a parallel ability to damage genetic material. As before, this model implied that cancer cells carry mutated genes.

One additional clue, even fainter, came from observations by the German biologist Theodor Boveri. In 1914, he had reported that the chromosomes of cancer cells were often jumbled in a general state of disarray. Since chromosomes were increasingly implicated as the repositories of a cell's genetic information, this too pointed to genetic damage as the driving force behind cancer.

In the end, it was not work on physical (radiation) carcinogens but on chemical ones that more dramatically advanced our understanding of the genetic basis of cancer and the

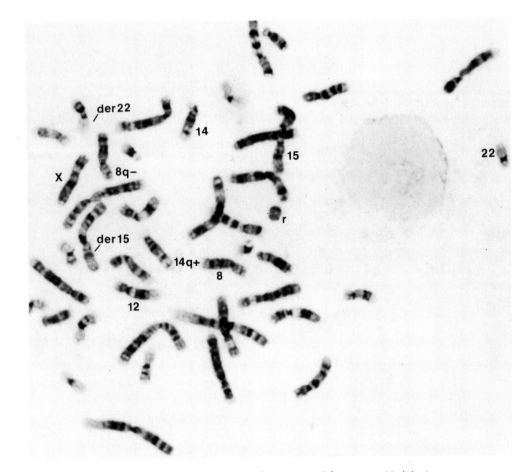

Chromosomes in a cancer cell often suffer a number of alterations. These, prepared from a non-Hodgkin's lymphoma, include a chromosome 8 with a shortened long arm (8q−); a chromosome 14 with a lengthened long arm (14q+); two derivatives of chromosomes 15 and 22 that have acquired extra material as a consequence of unidentified translocations; and a small, bizarre ring (r) chromosome, formed by joining the ends of a normally linear chromosome.

critical role of mutagenesis in this process. Carcinogenic chemicals had been known since the pioneering work in Japan of Katsusaburo Yamagiwa and Koichi Ichikawa, who showed in 1918 that skin cancers can be induced on rabbit ears by repeated applications of coal tar. In the following three decades, dozens of potently carcinogenic chemicals, including discrete components of coal tar, had been identified and isolated.

How, then, could these carcinogens elicit cancer? By the late 1940s, the genetic material was known to be carried by the DNA molecules present in the cell's chromosomes. If carcinogens acted by damaging genes, then the target of carcinogens was no longer elusive: it was precisely the DNA carried in the nuclei of cells. DNA, being of complex chemical structure, could have its structure altered by direct reaction with carcinogens. (Indeed, as early as the 1940s, several types of carcinogenic molecules had been found tightly bound to the DNA molecules of carcinogen-treated cells.) Because genetic information was encoded in this DNA structure, gene mutation might ensue.

CARCINOGENS AS MUTAGENS

This model of carcinogen-induced mutations received its most extensive test from Professor Bruce Ames, a microbiologist at the University of California in Berkeley. While it was known that some chemicals induce mutations unusually potently and others do so only weakly, a reliable, straightforward method of quantitating

this mutagenicity was lacking. The few tests available for measuring mutagenicity in mammalian cells were far too cumbersome, for a number of technical reasons. Ames decided instead to measure the ability of candidate mutagens to induce genetic damage in *Salmonella typhimurium*, the bacterium responsible for paratyphoid fever. Detecting mutant bacterial genes was far quicker and cheaper than searching for mutant genes in mammalian cells.

Implicit in Ames's test was the assumption that the genes of *Salmonella* bacteria serve as good models of mammalian genes. Both bacterial and mammalian cells use DNA as their genetic material, and both rely on a common genetic code in the DNA to specify the structures of their proteins. By measuring chemically induced mutations in a bacterial target gene (specifically, a gene controlling the metabolism of the amino acid histidine), Ames hoped to predict the response of genes in mammalian cells to these same chemicals.

Ames's strategy was to add test compounds to *Salmonella* and screen the bacterial populations for the occasional mutant colonies arising in response to these chemical treatments. Since up to 100 million *Salmonella* bacteria can be grown per petri dish, Ames could detect rare mutations that affected only one in a million bacteria.

But how could a mutant present as a single bacterium amid a million others be detected in culture? Ames designed his test so that the unmutated bacteria on the dish—the vast majority—were unable to grow when the amino acid histidine was omitted from the nutrient medium. However, the rare bacterial cell that sustained a mutation in one of its histidine-metabolizing genes could replicate prolifically, doubling every 30 to 40 minutes to yield a colony of descendants that was visible to the naked eye only 10 to 15 hours later. Such a technique requires no complicated measuring equipment, only the human eye. The more colonies counted, the more mutations attributable to the carcinogen previously applied to the culture. Ames could introduce carcinogens at various doses into a petri dish of *Salmonella* and, if all went well, count bacterial colonies after an overnight incubation. But the bacteria have one major disadvantage: they cannot metabolize many chemical compounds in the same way mammalian cells do. How could this problem be overcome?

THE AMES TEST REFINED

As the work of James and Elizabeth Miller had shown a decade earlier, the chemical structure of many carcinogenic molecules does not allow them to be mutagenic in the form in which they initially enter the cell. Instead, many known carcinogens are metabolically converted into highly reactive compounds only *within* cells. This metabolic activation into potent mutagens is carried out, ironically, by enzymes that the normal cell uses to neutralize various toxic compounds. In the absence of such metabolic activation, a potentially carcinogenic molecule will remain unreactive and therefore unable to alter biochemical targets like DNA.

Chemical mutagenesis in mammalian cells (and possible associated carcinogenesis) is often a two-step affair. First, a cell chemically alters an inert "pro-mutagen"; only then can the re-

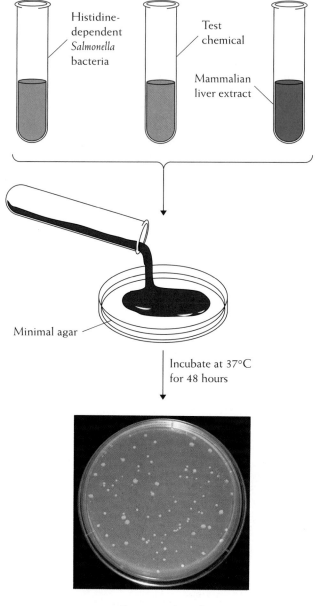

The Ames test demonstrates whether a given test chemical, when metabolized by the liver extract, becomes a potent mutagen.

sultant mutagen react directly with DNA, altering its chemical structure and thus its information content. Because bacterial cells lack this ability to activate pro-mutagens metabolically, Ames added a rat liver extract to the bacterial plates in which his assay was to be performed. The enzymes present in this liver preparation, acting as if they were in an intact mammalian cell, could modify many pro-mutagens. Activated by the liver enzyme slurry, these altered

Nature's Carcinogens

Bruce Ames, developer of the Ames test, evoked enormous controversy in the late 1980s by arguing that our society's obsession with trace-chemical pollutants in the water supply and man-made pesticide contaminants in fruits and vegetables has little rational basis. Using the Ames mutagen test and animal toxicity–carcinogenicity tests, he and others have screened extracts from a wide variety of plants and detected unexpectedly high levels of toxic, mutagenic chemical compounds among their natural constituents. These natural toxins may have evolved to protect the plants from insect predators; some of the natural pesticides may incidentally be carcinogenic for humans. For example, a recently bred strain of pest-resistant celery was found by Ames to contain 10 times more mutagens than its insect-susceptible progenitor. By Ames's calculation, the mass of natural pesticides consumed in our diet every day is as much as 10,000 times higher than the daily residue of man-made pesticides; these natural compounds, he argues, are as carcinogenic as those inadvertently introduced into the food chain through the use of agricultural chemicals. He calculates that the carcinogenic hazard of a glass of apple juice contaminated with the now-banned Alar (a chemical used to prevent premature ripening of apples) is 1/18th that of a peanut butter sandwich (having traces of the natural mold aflatoxin), 1/50th that of a mushroom, or 1/1000th that of a glass of beer (containing alcohol and natural fermentation products).

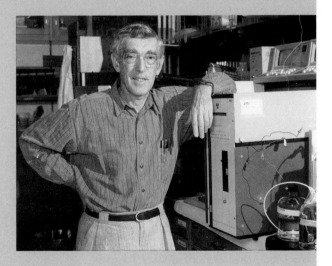

Bruce Ames.

Some Environmental Agents Implicated in Human Cancer Causation

AGENT	TARGET ORGAN FOR TUMORS
Aflatoxin (peanut mold)	Liver
Alcohol	Pharynx, larynx, esophagus, liver, (breast?)
Asbestos	Pleura of lung
X rays	Bone marrow (leukemia)
Sunlight (UV)	Skin
Aniline dyes	Bladder
Chewing tobacco	Mouth
Tobacco smoke	Mouth, lung, bladder, esophagus, pancreas
Hepatitis B virus (HBV)	Liver
Human T-cell leukemia virus	Thymus–spleen (leukemias)
Epstein-Barr virus	Bone marrow (lymphoma), nasopharynx
Human papilloma viruses	Uterine cervix

molecules could diffuse into the bacterial cells and interact there with the bacterial target gene.

In 1975, Ames published the first of the studies in which he used his bacterial test to measure the mutagenic potency of a diverse group of chemicals, including carcinogens known from previous trials in laboratory rodents. Various doses of candidate compounds had been fed to groups of 20 to 100 rats over a period of one to two years, making it possible to calculate the amount required to induce cancer in 50 percent of the animals. The carcinogenic potencies of test chemicals differed widely—from the aflatoxin made by a mold growing on peanuts, able to induce cancer in

50 percent of mice at daily doses as low as one microgram, to saccharin, which requires a millionfold higher dose to elicit a similar number of tumors. (These quantities are proportional to a teaspoonful versus a truckload.)

Ames's work yielded a striking correlation. Compounds that were known to be potent carcinogens were generally found to be potent mutagens; those that were weak carcinogens demonstrated reduced ability to induce mutations. Although we now know that many compounds do not follow this correlation, the many successes of the Ames test and its dramatic correlation between mutagenicity and carcinogenicity had widespread influence. At the purely technical level, the test could be adapted to screen candidate compounds of unknown carcinogenicity for their mutagenic potency. Any chemical that registered strongly in this test, which is at least a hundredfold cheaper and quicker than large-scale animal testing, became a suspected carcinogen, potentially dangerous to exposed human beings.

A UNIFIED THEORY EMERGES

These findings also encouraged those researchers who argued that chemical carcinogens act directly through their mutagenic ability. Their

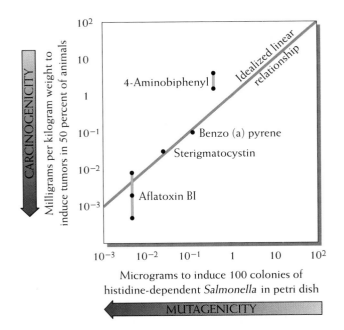

The mutagenic potency of four test compounds (horizontal axis) plotted against their carcinogenic potency when fed to laboratory rodents (vertical axis).

theoretical model was straightforward: carcinogens enter various tissues throughout the body; become activated, once within the cells, into potent mutagens; and induce mutations in critical target genes. These mutated genes direct the cells in which they reside to grow abnormally, and the cells' descendants appear months or years later as a tumor. Absent from this model were any predictions about the nature of the target genes or how, in mutant form, they could program malignant cell growth. Nevertheless, the door now opened to a new and simplified view of cancer's origins that combined these results with the demonstration by tumor virologists that a small number of viral oncogenes suffices to convert a normal cell into a tumor cell.

One could now speculate that a small number of specific genes native to the cell might, following alteration by mutagenic carcinogens, also initiate cancer. Once damaged and mutated by carcinogens, the altered versions of these so-called cancer genes could orchestrate abnormal cell growth by mechanisms analogous to those of oncogenes brought into cells by infecting tumor viruses.

This model formed the basis of our modern molecular theory of cancer. But in 1975 it was at best a vague and hardly conclusive description of how cancer begins. Its main fault was obvious: the identity of these cellular genes was elusive; indeed, their very existence was unproven. Were the virogenes—oncogenes of Huebner and Todaro the targets of carcinogens? Were other, cell-associated genes the important substrate for mutagen action? These puzzles have now been solved, as we shall see in the pages that follow.

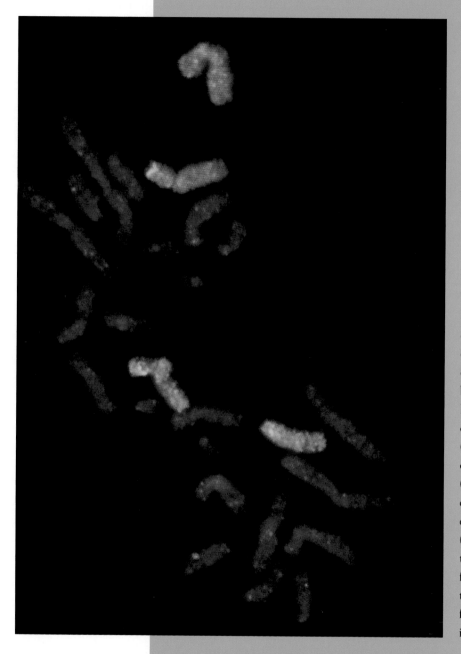

With a new technology, chromosomes from human cells are "painted" distinctive colors to reveal exchanges of material (translocations) between chromosomes. Here a normal chromosome 7 is all red (top); a normal chromosome 12 is all green (bottom). The two products of translocations between chromosomes 7 and 12 (middle) show green and red tips, respectively. Such findings direct investigators to certain chromosomes to find the specific genes involved in cancer.

4

THE GENETIC ELEMENTS GOVERNING CANCER: PROTO-ONCOGENES

M any of the observed associations between cancers and the diverse factors cited in the preceding chapter can be subsumed in a genetic theory of carcinogenesis, positing that cancers arise through a series of mutations affecting somatic cells during the lifetime of the organism, sometimes abetted by one or more inherited mutations. The somatically acquired mutations may result from exposure to a variety of environmental factors, such as certain chemicals or ionizing radiation; errors occurring naturally during duplication of cellular DNA; or the joining of viral genes to host chromosomes.

A unified genetic theory of cancer raises important questions about human health: How can mutations that predispose to cancer be prevented? Can they be detected early? Or combated therapeutically? Before such practical issues can be addressed, it is crucial to answer a number of more fundamental questions: What are the specific cellular genes that serve as targets for oncogenic mutations? What kinds of mutations occur? What are the normal functions of the affected genes? What are the biological consequences of the mutations?

EARLY APPROACHES: INSPECTION OF CHROMOSOMES

Concrete ideas about the genetic basis of cancer began to take hold in the 1950s and 1960s, following the revelation that genes are composed of DNA but before the advent of recombinant DNA techniques that simplified the isolation of genes from complex organisms. During this period, there were only two plausible experimental approaches to the genes that might be implicated in cancer. One was to inspect chromosomes from tumor cells in a conventional light microscope. Studies of this relatively crude type demonstrated that the genetic content of cancer cells was often abnormal: some chromosomes were present in three or four copies, rather than the usual two, and others had been rearranged by deletion, inversion of segments, or exchange of material between chromosomes.

The exchanges (translocations) assumed particular importance when some were recognized to occur regularly in certain types of cancers. For example, an abnormal chromosome known as the Philadelphia chromosome (Ph1), derived from an exchange between chromosomes 9 and 22, is found almost universally in tumor cells from patients with chronic myeloid leukemia. Such regularity strongly implies that genes affected by the translocations might be instrumental in the genesis of the associated tumors. But no technique available for microscopic inspection of disordered chromosomes permits identification of the affected genes. Since each chromosome is likely to contain 2000 to 10,000 genes and, for most chromosomes, less than 100 of these have been isolated and assigned approximate positions on the map of the human genome, we have little chance of predicting the genes at the joining points of translocated chromosomes without further information.

EARLY APPROACHES: ONCOGENIC VIRUSES

A second method for studying the genetic basis of cancer, described in the last chapter, made it possible to assign oncogenic potential to specific genes. This was the use of cancer-causing viruses from experimental animals. Recall that while most animal viruses destroy the cells they infect, several types of viruses are able to establish a long-term infection, in which the cell is not killed. These stable virus–host-cell interactions depend upon perpetuating the viral genetic information in the cell, usually by direct insertion into cellular chromosomes.

Acquisition of viral genes does not necessarily cause production of virus particles, and the host cell may not be incapacitated; rather, it may now have the heightened growth properties characteristic of a cancer cell, in the event that the viral genes issue growth-stimulating instructions. Such viruses are attractive tools for the study of cancer. Carrying relatively few genes—in some cases less than five, in others up to a hundred—these viruses are nevertheless able to convert a normal animal cell to a cancer cell within days. The situation contrasts sharply with naturally occurring human cancers, which develop over years as the result of a small number of altered genes that are difficult to identify among a pool of 50,000 to 100,000 candidate genes.

Cancer viruses have been isolated from virtually every type of vertebrate animal, induce a wide variety of tumors, and belong to several virus types. Most important for this chapter are the retroviruses, in which the genes are composed of RNA, but there are also four types of DNA tumor viruses: the polyomaviruses, the papillomaviruses, the adenoviruses, and the herpesviruses. The history of cancer research has been deeply affected by the experimental advantages and disadvantages of working with each of these viruses. Retroviruses and polyomaviruses have received most of the attention, in part because they have the smallest genomes, but also because many carry one or two genes that have specific cancer-inducing properties: so-called viral oncogenes. Like cellular genes, these viral genes are subject to mutations, and mutations that impair the genes also reduce or eliminate the ability of the viruses to cause cancer. One great advantage of the retroviruses and polyomaviruses was the early isolation of viral mutants that fail to cause tumors or lack the capacity to transform cells in culture. In each case, the defects in a virus could be assigned to a specific gene present in the viral genome. By implicating individual viral genes in the cancer-causing (oncogenic) process, these mutants provided a crucial starting point both for dissection of virus-induced cancers and for formulating the concept of an oncogene—a gene that dominates the behavior of the cell in which it acts, helping to convert the cell to a cancerous state.

THE SRC GENE OF ROUS SARCOMA VIRUS

Certain mutations in the viral genome do not destroy the transforming (oncogenic) function outright, but affect it more subtly. A group of such mutants of Rous sarcoma virus (RSV) has proved highly useful for research. Termed temperature-sensitive, these mutant viruses have the striking characteristic of failing to transform infected cells when the cells are grown at an elevated temperature, although they remain able to transform the same cells at a lower temperature. The continued ability of the mu-

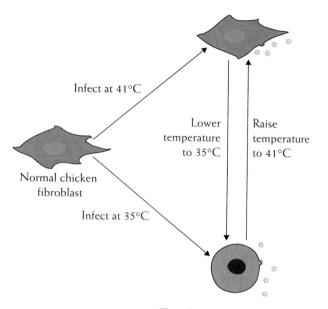

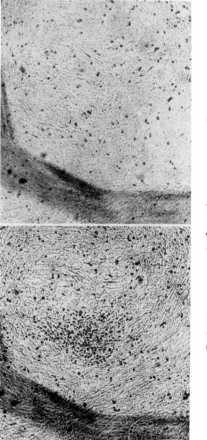

Infected;
not transformed

41°C

35°C

Infected;
transformed
(note focus)

Chicken fibroblasts infected by a temperature-sensitive mutant of Rous sarcoma virus (RSV) are transformed at 35°C but not at 41°C, yet produce new virus particles at both temperatures. The photograph at right shows the changes in cell shape that occur within a few hours after shifting the temperature up or down.

tant viruses to multiply normally in infected cells at either temperature, however, implies that the altered gene is not required for some step in the ordinary viral replication process, such as entry into the cell or expression of viral genes. When cells infected and transformed by such mutants at the lower temperature are shifted to the higher temperature, they lose their cancerous properties; conversely, cells initially infected at the higher temperature become transformed when the temperature is lowered.

Taken together, these observations imply that RSV has at least one gene whose protein product is continuously required to maintain cell transformation but is completely dispensable for viral growth. This viral gene—v-src—carries, in these mutants, nucleotide sequence changes that account for the temperature sensitivity of its transforming ability. It was presumed (and later demonstrated) that the v-src gene encodes a protein with a growth-perturbing function. Temperature-sensitive mutations of the v-src gene alter the structure of this

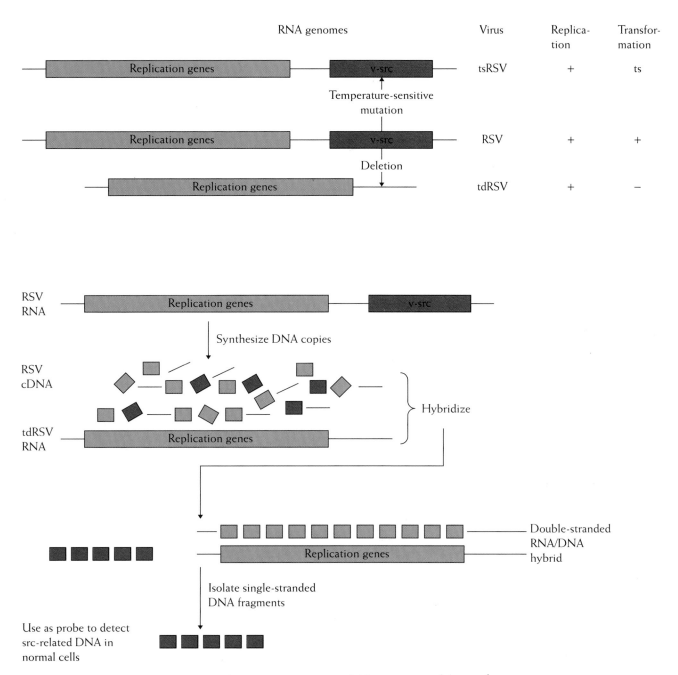

RNA genomes	Virus	Replication	Transformation

The diagram shows RNA genomes labeled with Replication genes and v-src regions:

- Replication genes | v-src — tsRSV — + — ts
  - Temperature-sensitive mutation
- Replication genes | v-src — RSV — + — +
  - Deletion
- Replication genes — tdRSV — + — −

RSV RNA: Replication genes | v-src

Synthesize DNA copies

RSV cDNA

tdRSV RNA: Replication genes

Hybridize

Replication genes — Double-stranded RNA/DNA hybrid

Isolate single-stranded DNA fragments

Use as probe to detect src-related DNA in normal cells

Genomes of wild-type RSV and strains with temperature-sensitive and deletion mutants of the transforming region. A DNA probe for the transforming (src) region of the RSV genome was prepared by making short DNA copies of RSV RNA, then removing irrelevant pieces, which form hybrids with complementary RNA from the tdRSV deletion mutant.

protein so that it loses activity when the temperature rises above a certain level and regains it when the temperature falls.

That temperature-sensitive transformation mutants of RSV multiply normally at both high and low temperatures suggested that RSV carries, in fact, two kinds of genes in its small genome. One set (comprising, as it turned out, only the single gene v-src) is required for transformation but is irrelevant for growth of the virus. Another set, essential for virus growth, is perhaps dispensable for transformation. This idea received strong confirmation from another type of RSV mutant that, by deletion, lacks part or all of the v-src gene. Such mutants, unable to manufacture v-src protein in any form, cannot transform cells at any temperature; but they retain the genes necessary to replicate normally and make new virus particles in infected cells.

The differences between the oncogenic genome of normal RSV and the nononcogenic genome of most deletion mutants could be mapped to a region in the viral genome of about 2000 nucleotides. Indeed, the size and position of these v-src inactivating deletions nearly coincide with those of the src gene; thus the mutants added a vital feature to the map of the RSV genome. But these deletion mutants afforded another, more practical benefit: they made it possible to isolate a small DNA segment corresponding to the src gene that could be used as a "probe" for detecting the presence or absence of src gene copies in infected or uninfected cells. This experimental strategy soon led to a remarkable discovery that fundamentally changed the study of cancer.

THE DISCOVERY OF C-SRC AND OTHER PROTO-ONCOGENES

The origins of most viral genes are obscured by the ability of viruses to evolve independently of the organisms they infect. To whatever extent some viral genes may initially have arisen from cellular antecedents, that relationship is usually no longer apparent. Thus, it is rare to find viral genes or their close relatives in cells not known to have been previously infected. One class of viruses, however, provides important exceptions to this rule.

It has been recognized for many years that retroviruses have unusual relationships with their host species. As the last chapter noted, many and perhaps all vertebrate animals, including humans, inherit genes related to retroviral genes and transmit them to their progeny. Because these genes are usually arranged in the same order as in infectious retroviral genomes, most were probably introduced into the germ cells of vertebrates by infection at some point in the past. These so-called endogenous proviruses could, in theory, have included viral oncogenes. In the mid-1970s, researchers sought to test the hypothesis that cancer arises when environmental agents induce the expression of viral oncogenes like v-src that reside in normal chromosomes as components of inherited proviruses (see Chapter 3).

One way to test this idea was to use the molecular probe for the v-src gene to determine whether v-src was present in the DNA of normal chickens. Uninfected chickens did in-

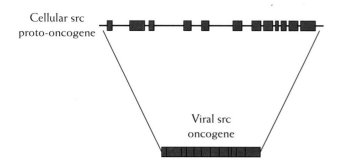

The viral oncogene of RSV (v-src) is derived from many exons of the c-src proto-oncogenes.

herit nucleotide sequences very closely related to the RSV src oncogene. But additional experiments disclosed that these sequences were not, as had been speculated, acquired as part of a germline infection that led to the establishment of an endogenous provirus. The v-src-related sequences were not positioned within or near other retroviral genes in chicken chromosomes; more surprisingly, they could be found in many kinds of birds—quail, ducks, even emus—and were later detected in the genomes of all vertebrate orders and many other metazoans, including worms, insects, and sponges. This widespread presence of v-src-related DNA contrasts with the pattern of an endogenous provirus, which will not be found in related species that do not descend from a common infected ancestor; endogenous proviruses closely related to RSV could, in fact, be found only in chickens. The src-like sequences in normal cells were therefore proposed to constitute a cellular gene, called c-src. As expected of a cellular gene, its coding sequences are segmented into exons, separated by introns (retrovirus genes usually lack introns).

What, then, is the relationship between the v-src oncogene and the c-src gene that resides in the genome of normal chickens and, for that matter, apparently in the genomes of all animals? The answer, worked out in the following years, was that the viral src gene descends directly from a c-src cellular antecedent. A precursor of Rous sarcoma virus that was able to replicate but unable to transform cells seems to have picked up a copy of c-src during infection of a chicken cell. The resulting virus, which we term RSV, then exploited its acquired gene to transform subsequently infected cells. This astounding finding testified dramatically to the versatility of retroviruses. But why was such a gene, with cancer-causing potential, present in a host-cell genome in the first place? The remarkable evolutionary conservation of c-src implied that the gene is not intrinsically harmful but actually must confer some essential benefit. After all, this gene has been conserved in virtually unaltered form since the time—a billion years ago—when the common ancestor to all modern metazoans first appeared.

If c-src is a crucial and beneficial gene, however, why does its close relative v-src cause tumors and transform cells after RSV infection? New techniques that permitted careful comparisons of v-src and c-src showed that the genes differ in at least two important ways. Under the control of strong viral signals, v-src produces much more src protein in RSV-infected cells than is found in normal cells expressing c-src; a chicken fibroblast transformed by RSV produces about 50 times more src RNA and protein than an uninfected fibroblast containing only the c-src gene. Also, the protein-coding sequence of v-src has been changed by several mutations that presumably occurred during or after the acquisition of src sequences by a viral genome. The resulting structurally altered v-src protein, unlike the c-src precursor protein, is competent to transform cells even when produced in small amounts. The acquisition of the src gene by the ancestor of RSV was accompanied, in short, by quantitative and qualitative effects, both of which help to make the gene oncogenic.

The discovery of c-src showed unambiguously that the genome of a normal cell harbors at least one gene that can be activated into a potent oncogene under certain (admittedly very special) circumstances—in this case, when captured by a retrovirus. Such a gene, normal but possessing latent carcinogenic powers, was termed a proto-oncogene to suggest this potential without prejudging its usual function.

Recall from Chapter 3 that a series of carcinogenic chemicals had been thought to in-

Retrovirus	Genome	Virus replication	Transformation of cells in culture	Tumor induction
RSV	v-src	+	+	Sarcomas (fast)
ALV		+	–	B-cell lymphomas and erythroleukemias (slow)
MC29	v-myc	–	+	Myeloid leukemias (fast)
MLV		+	–	T-cell lymphomas (slow)
Abelson-MLV	v-abl	–	+	B-cell lymphomas (fast)
Ha-MSV	v-Ha-ras	–	+	Sarcomas (fast)
MMTV		+	–	Breast carcinomas (slow)

A comparison of the ability of various retroviruses, with and without viral oncogenes, to multiply, to transform cells, and to induce cancers in animals.

Retroviral Oncogenes

Viral Oncogene (v-onc)	Prototype Virus	Species of Origin
src	Rous sarcoma virus	Chicken
yes	Yamaguchi 73 sarcoma virus	Chicken
myc	Myelocytomatosis-29 virus	Chicken
erbA	Avian erythroblastosis virus	Chicken
erbB	Avian erythroblastosis virus	Chicken
jun	Avian sarcoma virus 17	Chicken
rel	Reticuloendotheliosis virus, strain T	Turkey
mos	Moloney murine sarcoma virus	Mouse
abl	Abelson murine leukemia virus	Mouse
raf	Murine sarcoma virus 3611	Mouse
fos	Mouse (osteo) sarcoma virus	Mouse
Ha-ras	Harvey murine sarcoma virus	Rat
Ki-ras	Kirsten murine sarcoma virus	Rat
fms	Susan McDonough feline sarcoma virus	Cat
kit	Hardy-Zuckerman 4 feline sarcoma virus	Cat
sis	Simian sarcoma virus	Woolly monkey

duce cancer by mutating specific cellular target genes. While an attractive theory, it lacked one critical ingredient: no one knew the nature or identity of these genes—until the discovery of c-src revealed an excellent candidate.

The c-src gene took on greater significance when it was recognized that many other retroviruses carry oncogenes, often fundamentally different from v-src. Each of these genes is also derived from a distinct, normal cellular precursor. One prominent example is the gene present in MC29 virus, an agent of myeloid leukemia in chickens. This virus bears an oncogene, v-myc, that was traced to its progenitor gene, c-myc, in normal chicken DNA. Two tumor-inducing viruses of rodents, the Harvey and Kirsten strains of murine sarcoma virus, likewise contain related viral oncogenes, v-Ha-ras and v-Ki-ras, that originated from two cellular genes, now known as c-Ha-ras and c-Ki-ras. (Several other viral oncogenes derived from normal cellular genes are listed in the table on page 75.) Extension of the v-src paradigm to more than 20 other retroviral oncogenes dramatically expanded the roster of cellular genes that, on the one hand, had served as precursors to virus-borne oncogenes and, on the other, might potentially serve as targets for alteration and activation by mutagenic agents. As we shall soon describe, proto-oncogenes can be discovered by means other than the study of retroviruses; they serve diverse biochemical functions in the control of normal cell growth and development; and they can undergo a variety of mutations that convert them to dominant genes capable of inducing cancers in the absence of viruses.

PROVIRAL ACTIVATION OF PROTO-ONCOGENES

Proto-oncogenes, it was clear, can induce cancer when they are captured and subverted by retroviruses, but this raised an equally provocative issue: Could these genes induce cancer while still residing in their normal chromosomal site? One of the first indications that a proto-oncogene can indeed be mutated in its native chromosomal context emerged from attempts to solve another mystery about retroviruses. Although the most potent of the oncogenic retroviruses carry viral oncogenes like v-src, derived from cellular proto-oncogenes, many other retroviruses do not carry their own oncogenes but are nevertheless able to induce

tumors in susceptible animals. These oncogene-free retroviruses take a relatively long time—months rather than days or weeks—to cause tumors, a delay suggesting that additional, rare events, perhaps even multiple events, must also occur in the cohort of infected cells to produce a tumor. If the requisite events took place within a single cell, the long interval between infection and the appearance of a tumor could in part reflect the time required for that cell to produce a large number of descendant cancer cells: a clonal tumor population. In contrast, infection by an oncogene-bearing virus like RSV can immediately convert most or all of the cells it infects into cancer cells in a single step, rapidly forming a polyclonal tumor composed of millions of independently infected cells.

What kinds of rare events might cause oncogenic changes in infected cells? Reconsider briefly a few aspects of the retrovirus growth cycle. In the initial stages of infection, the RNA genome present in a retrovirus particle is copied into DNA by a viral enzyme called reverse transcriptase. Once synthesized, the viral DNA molecule is transported into the nucleus and inserted as a provirus into the chromosomes of the host cell randomly at any one of millions of available sites. In the process, a region of host-chromosomal DNA is cut and the viral DNA genome is swiftly joined to the cut ends, so that the provirus is integrated within the host's chromosome. Might a retrovirus lacking its own oncogenes occasionally tuck its provirus into the host chromosomes next to a proto-oncogene? Proviruses are known to possess signals for the regulation of their own (viral) genes; might such signals be transmitted along the chromosomes to the proto-oncogene, compelling it to produce larger than normal amounts of RNA and protein? In this way, a proto-oncogene could be activated without being removed from the chromosome.

These ideas were first validated by the study of a chicken leukosis virus that causes lymphomas arising from B lymphocytes although it lacks its own oncogene. Examination of cellular DNA from many independently arising tumors showed that despite the tendency of proviruses to integrate randomly throughout the host-cell genome, the DNA of all these tumor cells displayed a proviral insertion at virtually the same chromosomal location. Amazingly and invariably, proviruses in the lymphoma cells were within or adjacent to the c-myc gene, the proto-oncogenic forebear of the v-myc oncogene in MC29 virus. As anticipated, the concentrations of c-myc messenger RNA and protein are abnormally high in these tumor cells, because viral regulatory signals influence transcription of the adjacent c-myc gene. Subsequent work, presented below, supports the notion that a variety of changes in the c-myc gene can deregulate its expression and thereby contribute to oncogenesis in many cell types and many species, including human beings.

Studies of many other retroviruses that cause tumors without the aid of viral onco-

Insertions of retroviral DNA can increase the production of RNA and protein by a proto-oncogene (top), turn on a previously silent proto-oncogene (center), or cause the production of an abnormal (e.g., truncated) protein (bottom).

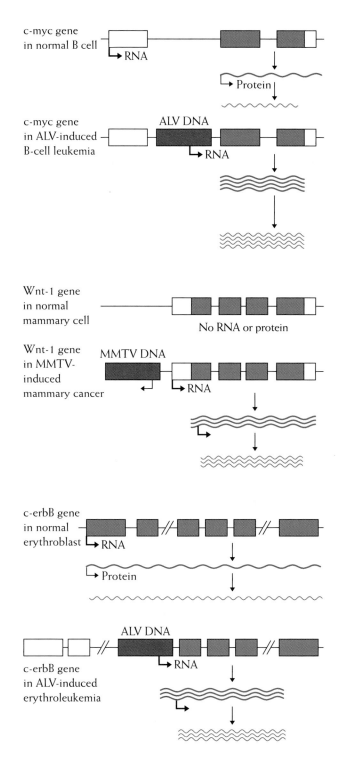

genes have suggested that an early step in tumorigenesis is activation of a proto-oncogene by a proviral insertion mutation. Often the activated gene is c-myc, but in many situations other known proto-oncogenes are involved. For instance, when chicken leukosis viruses induce erythroleukemia (a leukemia of red-blood-cell precursors) rather than B-cell lymphoma, the affected gene is c-erbB, the cellular homolog of the v-erbB oncogene carried by avian erythroleukemia virus. But oncogene-free retroviruses sometimes initiate tumorigenesis by inserting their proviruses next to genes previously unknown. This has led to the discovery of entirely novel proto-oncogenes, now almost as numerous as those discovered as precursors of viral oncogenes. The mouse mammary tumor virus, for example, can activate at least five cellular genes by inserting its proviral DNA next to them at their various chromosomal locations. Although none of these genes has ever been encountered as a viral oncogene in a naturally occurring retrovirus, there is strong evidence that these genes play direct roles in carcinogenesis when they are inappropriately expressed in mammary epithelial cells.

Retroviruses have thus provided two general methods for discovering cellular proto-oncogenes: tracing viral oncogenes to their cellular origins and analyzing DNA in virus-induced tumors for cellular genes that may be activated by adjacent proviruses. More than 50 proto-oncogenes have been identified by one route or the other, and several (such as c-myc and c-erbB) have been sighted both ways; as will become clear in later sections, these genes encode a wide variety of proteins that are active in many different steps in growth control

and differentiation. Additional approaches have been refined to discover still other proto-oncogenes and to determine which can be converted to oncogenes in human cancers.

GENE TRANSFER AND TRANSFORMING GENES

The most important of the additional methods for isolating oncogenes has been gene transfer into cultured cells. The introduction of one cell's DNA into another for the purpose of transferring genetic properties has been a staple in experimental biology since the 1940s, when it was used to confer traits of one bacterium upon another, providing the first tangible evidence that genetic information is carried in DNA molecules. In subsequent years, gene

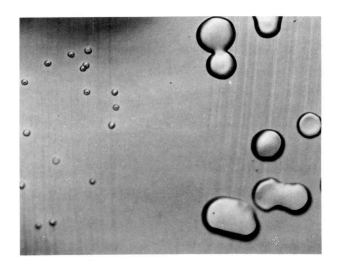

In classical experiments by Avery, Macleod, and McCarty, DNA was shown to be the factor from encapsulated bacteria that converts noncapsular strains (left) to a capsular form (right).

transfer has been achieved in many settings: from one type of cultured animal cell to another; from several kinds of viruses to host cells; from a wide range of organisms to bacterial or yeast cells for purposes of molecular cloning; and from various sources to fertilized mouse eggs to produce new breeds of permanently altered, transgenic mice, as we will see later in this chapter. The proto-oncogenes discovered through retrovirology appeared, as mentioned earlier, likely to be genes that might also be mutated by carcinogenic chemicals. Could gene transfer be used to detect mutated oncogenes in the genomes of tumor cells that had been transformed by chemical carcinogens rather than retroviruses?

In the early 1970s, DNA prepared from RSV-transformed cells was introduced by gene transfer into normal recipient cells. The normal cells became transformed. This showed dramatically that the viral genetic information— specifically, its transforming gene(s)—was carried in the form of DNA molecules, as suspected. Such results, obtained with a viral oncogene, suggested that it might be possible to detect a *cellular* oncogene (that is, a mutated proto-oncogene) if it were transferred from a cancer cell into a recipient normal cell by this method. Like the v-src gene in an RSV provirus, a cellular oncogene might represent a single gene copy amid a vast excess of other cellular DNA. As before, the important criteria for recipient cells are an ability to take up foreign DNA efficiently and to respond to any introduced oncogene by an easily recognized change in behavior; in this case, conversion to a transformed state. Most experiments were done with a standard line of mouse fibroblasts

from the National Institutes of Health (NIH3T3 cells).

The first reported successes with this new method for seeking oncogenes used DNA from mouse cells that had been transformed by exposure to chemical carcinogens. The observed ability of DNA extracted from such cells to transform recipient NIH3T3 cells strongly implied that at least one mutated gene was carried in the chemically transformed cells and could be transferred to the recipient cells. In principle, that oncogene could be isolated and identified.

Shortly thereafter, DNA samples from a surprisingly wide variety of human cancers were found to induce transformation of NIH3T3 cells, prompting an intensive hunt for the active oncogene(s) in several of these tumor-cell DNAs. When a combination of gene transfer and DNA cloning procedures made it possible to isolate a few such genes and inspect their nucleotide sequences, two surprises were encountered. First, most of the cellular oncogenes were immediately recognizable as versions of the c-Ha-ras or c-Ki-ras proto-oncogenes, the progenitors of retroviral oncogenes carried by strains of murine sarcoma virus. In other words, the same proto-oncogene could apparently be activated in rodents when captured by a retrovirus and in humans by nonviral means involving direct gene alteration, perhaps by mutagenic chemicals. Second, subtle differences distinguished the tumor-associated ras oncogenes from the corresponding proto-oncogenes found in normal human cells. Comparison revealed that each ras oncogene invariably contained a single nucleotide change (termed a point mutation) that altered

	1	2	3	4	5	6	7	8	9	10	11	12	13		188	189	
Normal human c-Ha-ras	Met	Thr	Glu	Tyr	Lys	Leu	Val	Val	Val	Gly	Ala	Gly	Gly		Leu	Ser	Amino acid
	ATG	ACG	GAA	TAT	AAG	CTG	GTG	GTG	GTG	GGC	GCC	GGC	GGT	.... CTC	TCC		Codon

↓

													GTC					Codon
Activated c-Ha-ras	Met	Thr	Glu	Tyr	Lys	Leu	Val	Val	Val	Gly	Ala	Val	Gly	.... Leu	Ser		Amino acid

The active Ha-ras oncogene often differs from the Ha-ras proto-oncogene by a single nucleotide change in the twelfth codon, causing an important alteration in the amino acid sequence of ras protein.

the amino acid sequence of the protein that it encoded. In different tumors these nucleotide substitutions often affected the same site in the gene, suggesting either that certain sites in the gene are especially mutable or that changes in certain regions of the protein are especially likely to create oncogenic function. In either case, it was apparent that oncogenes in human cancers that had arisen independently of viral infection were point-mutated versions of normal cellular proto-oncogenes.

These findings suggested, although they did not directly prove, that carcinogens indeed act as mutagens, inducing point mutations in critical target genes of the cells they enter. Some of these targets are ras proto-oncogenes, which are converted into potent oncogenes as a consequence of the mutations. The newly created ras oncogenes clearly issue instructions that are sufficient to force NIH3T3 cells (into which they have been introduced by gene transfer) to display transformed properties. Presumably, these oncogenes had similar effects in those cells in which the mutations originally occurred.

Through the use of oncogene transfer into NIH3T3 cells, it is now known that many human and experimental cancer cells also have single base substitutions in their c-Ha-ras, c-Ki-ras, or N-ras genes. (N-ras is a third member of the ras gene family, closely related to the other two and discovered through the use of the NIH3T3 cell assay.) Because these mutations almost always involve the twelfth, thirteenth, or sixty-first codon of the ras genes, it has been possible to devise simple biochemical tests for these common mutations by direct analysis of the DNA sequence. These tests show that as many as 90 percent of certain human tumors (pancreatic carcinomas, for example) have mutated ras genes in their DNA. Overall, about one-fourth of human cancers carry mutant ras alleles.

In both experimental and human cancers, genes other than members of the ras family may also undergo mutations that are detected by the NIH3T3 cell assay. A few of these, like the first two ras genes, were already known as progenitors of retroviral oncogenes; others, like N-ras, were newly discovered, albeit usu-

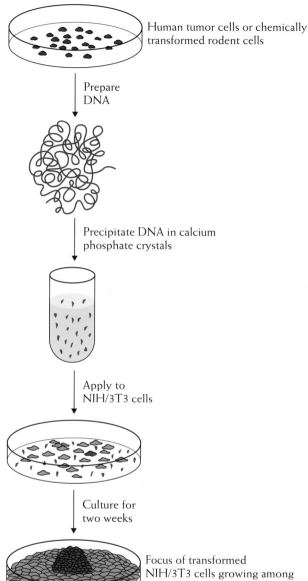

Human tumor cells or chemically transformed rodent cells

Prepare DNA

Precipitate DNA in calcium phosphate crystals

Apply to NIH/3T3 cells

Culture for two weeks

Focus of transformed NIH/3T3 cells growing among untransformed cells

The presence of a transforming gene in chemically transformed mouse cells or human tumor cells could be demonstrated by preparing tumor cell DNA, transfecting it into NIH3T3 cells, and scanning for the appearance of transformed cells several weeks later.

ally related to previously identified proto-oncogenes. The DNA from neuroblastomas in chemically treated rats, for example, contains an NIH3T3-transforming gene called neu or erb B-2; the neu oncogene is a base substitution mutant of a proto-oncogene closely related (but not identical) to c-erbB, the precursor of the avian erythroblastosis virus oncogene, v-erbB. Other oncogenes that transform NIH3T3 cells were entirely novel when first discovered through the use of this assay. Finally, not all the oncogenes detected in the gene transfer assay show single nucleotide changes—some are grossly rearranged, with blocks of hundreds or thousands of nucleotides deleted and the remaining sequences fused with novel sequences originating elsewhere in the cellular genome. These large changes in DNA structure can have alternative effects upon encoded proteins: some may be truncated; others may become joined with protein segments from unrelated genes to form hybrid proteins. Both sorts of protein alterations can be shown to have oncogenic activity in the NIH3T3 cell assay.

Many oncogenes do not register in the NIH3T3 cell assay because they are unable to induce the formation of characteristic foci (colonies of transformed cells). It might be anticipated that some specialized oncogenes active in producing cancers only in cell lineages unrelated to fibroblasts would fail to transform NIH3T3 cells. Furthermore, unlike normal cells cultured directly from embryos or adult tissues, NIH3T3 cells have undergone changes, including mutations, that allow them to grow indefinitely in culture; some normal obstacle to sustained growth has already been breached in these cells, and they may be unable to respond to certain oncogenes that confer similar properties upon normal cells. Yet such oncogenes, among them those belonging to the myc family, may nonetheless play important roles in creating a cancer cell.

ONCOGENES AT TRANSLOCATION BREAKPOINTS

Gene transfer into NIH3T3 cells has usually failed to identify the genes directly affected by chromosomal abnormalities, although we recall that translocation chromosomes, visible genetic aberrations, gave early support to mutational theories of cancer. (In translocation, two arms from different chromosomes become joined.) It has been assumed in all cases that translocations bring two previously unlinked genes into proximity; one then causes inappropriate expression of the other, or the genes fuse to create a hybrid gene with novel oncogenic functions. If such ideas are correct, it is critically important to establish the identities of the gene sequences on both sides of the junction of the two chromosomes, a site known to geneticists as a breakpoint.

To identify genes at translocation breakpoints generally requires a combination of approaches: approximate mapping of genes on normal chromosomes, inspired guesswork, and tedious molecular cloning. Several steps, for instance, were required to arrive at a satisfactory explanation of the translocation chromosome Ph1 present in virtually all human mye-

loid leukemias. First it was shown that the Ph1 chromosome arose through fusion of a small piece of chromosome 9 to most of chromosome 22. Then the c-abl proto-oncogene, the progenitor of the v-abl oncogene of the Abelson mouse leukemia virus, was mapped to chromosome 9, near or at the point where the

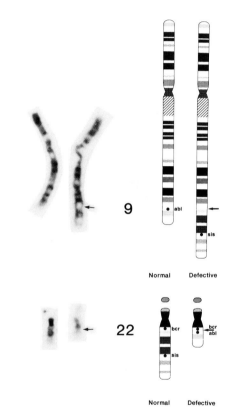

Photographs (left) and diagrams (right) of human chromosomes 9 and 22 and the products of the translocation that creates the Philadelphia chromosome (Ph1; lower right), commonly found in human leukemic cells, and its reciprocal. The translocation juxtaposes the genes bcr and abl, normally found on separate chromosomes.

breakage and fusion were thought to occur. Inspection of the detailed structure of c-abl in Ph1 chromosomes revealed that the gene was disrupted: the first segment of c-abl was missing and the remainder was fused to the middle of an unknown gene on chromosome 22 called bcr (for breakpoint cluster region). The Ph1 translocation results, then, in the formation of a hybrid gene (bcr-abl), which in turn makes a hybrid protein having novel, growth-promoting properties that predispose cells to become leukemic.

Translocation chromosomes like Ph1 occur repeatedly in certain types of cancers, especially leukemias. How might these occur? Chromosomes may continually exchange information with each other by random fusions, or translocations characteristic of certain types of tumors may represent the aberrant consequences of processes that normally occur in certain kinds of cells. Both of these ideas, in fact, may sometimes be true. Characteristic translocations occur regularly in cancerous growths of B and T lymphocytes, which make proteins required for immune functions—immunoglobulins (antibodies) and T-cell receptors (for recognition of antigens), respectively. To carry out their functions, B and T cells normally rearrange the DNA encoding these important proteins, using special mechanisms to cut and rejoin DNA within several chromosomal regions. In B-cell (and T-cell) lymphomas, it is common to find that part of an immunoglobulin (or T-cell receptor) gene has been joined to a proto-oncogene on a different chromosome. This implies that the machinery for normal antibody gene rearrangements has made an error, inadvertently creating a translocation chromosome and, as a consequence, an active oncogene. As with the Ph1 chromo-

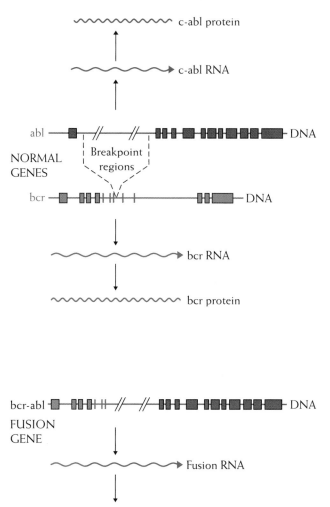

The fusion of bcr and abl genes in the Philadelphia chromosome creates a hybrid messenger RNA that encodes a hybrid protein with altered biochemical properties.

Translocated Proto-Oncogenes in Human Cancers

Chromosomal Partners	Known Genes at Breakpoints	Types of Cancers
9	c-abl	Chronic myeloid leukemia,
22	bcr	acute lymphocytic leukemia
8	c-myc	Burkitt's (B-cell) lymphoma
2, 14, or 22	Immunoglobulin gene	
18	bcl-2	Follicular B-cell lymphoma
14	Immunoglobulin gene	
15	pml	Acute promyelocytic leukemia
17	rar (retinoic acid receptor)	
1	PBX-1	Acute pre-B-cell leukemia
19	E2A	

some, such translocations have, in several cases, triggered successful searches for the proto-oncogenes that have been activated.

Consider the example of Burkitt's lymphoma, a B-cell tumor common in African children and associated with infection by the Epstein-Barr herpesvirus. In Burkitt's lymphoma, one arm of chromosome 8 is generally joined to one of three other chromosomes, at sites where three distinct immunoglobulin genes have been mapped. In each case, sequences that normally regulate expression of the immunoglobulin genes have been joined to the c-myc gene on chromosome 8, altering its pattern of expression: no longer governed by its own control elements, the c-myc gene appears to be placed under the control of a foreign regulator provided by one or another immunoglobulin gene. Since the c-myc proto-oncogene is known to have oncogenic potential (as a progenitor of the v-myc gene and as a target for insertional mutation by retroviruses), it is virtually certain that translocations of this type have a significant role in creating these lymphomas.

Patient guesswork, chromosomal mapping, and molecular cloning have allowed isolation of novel proto-oncogenes at translocation breakpoints, even when neither partner gene at the site of chromosomal fusion was previously known. Some of these newly discovered genes have proved clinically useful, especially in cancer diagnosis, as we will discuss in Chapter 8.

GENE AMPLIFICATION

Translocations are not the only kind of chromosomal abnormality frequently observed in cancer cells. Among the most dramatic are two others that suggest an inappropriate reduplication of one region of a chromosome, so that genes normally present in two copies per cell are found in dozens or even hundreds of copies, the consequence of gene amplification. The amount of DNA amplified into multiple copies can encompass one gene or a large region containing several genes. If the duplicated regions are linked end-to-end within a chromosome and attain sufficient length, they will distort the normal staining pattern of the chromosome as viewed under an ordinary light microscope; this distortion is characterized as a homogeneously staining region (HSR). Alternatively, the amplified DNA may be cut free of the chromosome and survive as tiny extrachromosomal circles of DNA known as double minute chromosomes (DMs), which can also be seen microscopically and may appear by the hundreds in each cell. Whether present as an HSR or as DMs, the amplified DNA can usually make both RNA and protein in amounts proportional to the elevated gene copy number. Thus the growth-stimulating activity of a proto-oncogene, amplified manyfold, may contribute to the creation of a cancer cell.

Among the first proto-oncogenes to be found amplified in tumor cells were c-myc and

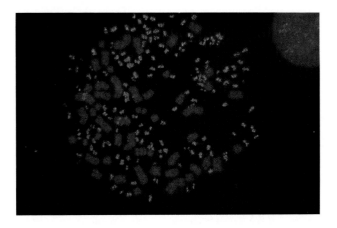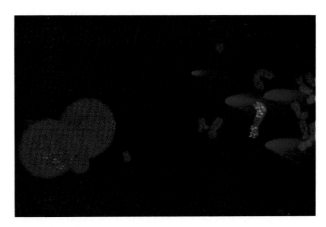

When DNA is inappropriately amplified, the amplified DNA can often be seen in stained chromosomes as pairs of tiny chromosomes called double minutes (left) or as expanded, homogeneously staining regions of chromosomes (right).

two close relatives, N-myc and L-myc; the latter two were unknown until detected by probes for c-myc (with which they share nucleotide sequences) in tumor cell lines carrying HSRs or DMs with grossly exaggerated numbers of gene copies. N-myc is characteristically amplified in the common childhood tumor neuroblastoma (hence N), whereas L-myc is more often amplified in small-cell carcinomas of the lung (hence L). Since gene amplification is relatively simple to measure, large numbers of neuroblastomas have been screened for N-myc copy number. The connection revealed between N-myc amplification and an unfavorable clinical prognosis is one criterion for claiming that an increased number of N-myc genes contributes to the oncogenic process (in other words, that N-myc is a proto-oncogene).

Examples of Proto-Oncogenes Amplified in Human Cancers

GENE	TUMOR TYPE
c-myc	Small-cell lung carcinoma Breast carcinoma
N-myc	Neuroblastoma Small-cell lung carcinoma
L-myc	Small-cell lung carcinoma
c-erbB	Epidermal carcinoma Glioblastoma
neu/erb-B2	Breast carcinoma

Compiling and Validating Proto-Oncogenes

Classification of genes as proto-oncogenes is ultimately based upon the conviction that mutant forms of these genes have a functional role in the development of cancer. Two kinds of evidence are generally advanced. First are the circumstantial factors: the finding of mutant versions of the gene in tumors, particularly in many tumors of the same type. The mutations affecting such genes—base substitutions, translocations, amplifications, or proviral insertions—are relatively rare, and the chance of a single cell sustaining such a mutation during a given cell cycle is probably no more than one in a million. For this reason, repeated occurrences of particular mutations in a series of independently arising tumors imply that they confer some special advantage upon the affected cell, most obviously the ability to grow more vigorously than unmutated neighboring cells.

Circumstantial arguments, of course, have their limits. Direct functional tests of oncogenic potential are ultimately preferable. One example is the gene transfer test described earlier, in which the powers of a candidate oncogene are tested by introducing it into a cultured cell, which then may respond by showing some neoplastic trait. In other cases a more elaborate strategy has been used: generation of transgenic mice. In this procedure, a candidate oncogene is introduced into the

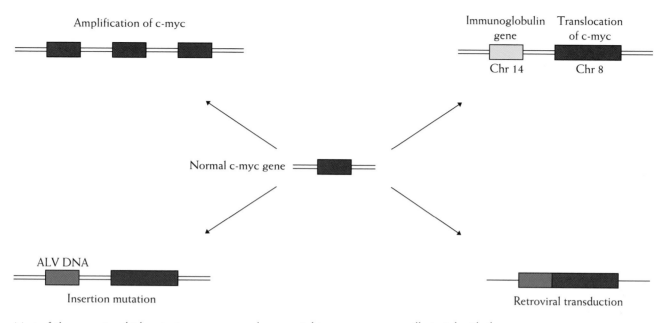

Amplification of c-myc

Immunoglobulin gene   Translocation of c-myc

Chr 14   Chr 8

Normal c-myc gene

ALV DNA

Insertion mutation

Retroviral transduction

Most of the ways in which a proto-oncogene can be converted to an oncogene are illustrated with the c-myc gene, which has been found to be activated by gene amplification, chromosomal translocation, retroviral transduction (forming a viral oncogene), and proviral insertion mutations.

germ line of mice by injecting a DNA clone of the gene into the nucleus of a fertilized egg. If the DNA is integrated into cells that produce the germ cells of the new animal, it will be inherited in a Mendelian fashion like other chromosomal genes, becoming a so-called transgene. By designing the DNA clone so that it is linked to transcriptional signals used preferentially in certain types of cells, expression of the resulting transgene can be targeted to specific tissues or organs. Such experiments demonstrate oncogenic activity powerfully, even in tissues that are difficult to propagate in cell culture, and they provide useful models for dissecting multiple phases of carcinogenesis (see Chapter 7).

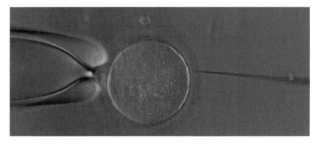

Injection of oncogene DNA into a fertilized egg (held stationary by the pipette on the left) is the first step in making a transgenic mouse that will develop tumors regularly.

Proteins Encoded by Proto-Oncogenes: The src Paradigm

To understand the functional attributes of normal and mutant versions of proto-oncogenes, we must recall that it is ultimately the protein products of oncogenes that do the work of transforming a cell. At this point, we are poised to consider the structure and biochemical activities of the kinds of proteins made by proto-oncogenes under normal conditions and after they have been mutated into oncogenes. In Chapter 6, we will attempt to integrate these proteins and their associated functions into a broader account of how cell growth is controlled.

Early investigation of the src oncogene of Rous sarcoma virus illustrates some of the difficulties and unexpected insights that have come from attempts to understand oncogenic proteins, especially in the era before molecular cloning. Until the mid-1970s, efforts to detect the v-src protein in RSV-transformed cells had met with failure. A very small fraction of the protein in such cells, less than one molecule in 100,000, is encoded by v-src, so some trick was required to separate the protein of interest from the vast amount of irrelevant cellular proteins. In principle, the best way to achieve this would be to derive antibodies that specifically recognize and bind the v-src protein, thereby permitting its precipitation and isolation from all other cellular proteins. But such antibodies were difficult to obtain; the most obvious source, serum from chickens bearing RSV-induced sarcomas, did not usually contain con-

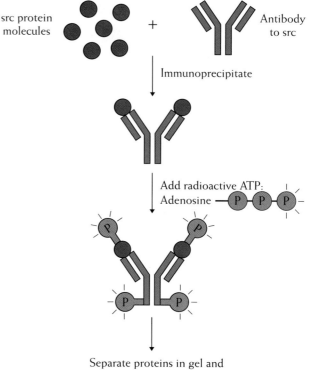

The protein kinase activity of src protein is observed by forming a complex with anti-src antibodies. The src kinase transfers radioactive phosphate from ATP to the heavy chain of the antibodies and to src protein itself. The radiolabeled proteins are then detected after separating the proteins by size with gel electrophoresis.

centrations of antibodies adequate for precipitating the v-src protein from virus-transformed cells.

This impasse was broken by an unorthodox strategy: RSV, which had been studied mostly in chickens, was introduced into rabbits. Although RSV will not usually grow in mammalian cells, it can occasionally enter and transform them. In fact, RSV can induce sarcomas in rabbits, well known as efficient producers of antibodies. These rabbit tumors frequently grow to a substantial size and then begin to shrink. Such tumor regression is often the sign of an active immune system that recognizes the tumor cells as foreign—in this case because they produce RSV-encoded protein—and succeeds in killing many of them. When sera (and thus antibodies) from tumor-bearing rabbits were mixed with extracts of RSV-infected chicken cells, they precipitated a protein of about 60,000 daltons in mass (slightly over 500 amino acids in length); this protein was not seen when the extracts were prepared from similar cells infected with an RSV mutant that lacked the v-src gene. By this criterion and many others, the protein was identified as the product that the v-src gene uses to transform cells. It was termed p60$^{\text{v-src}}$. As tests for viral src protein improved, it became possible to precipitate a similar but even less abundant protein of about 60,000 daltons from normal cells. This was the product of the c-src proto-oncogene, apparently used by the cell for its normal physiological functions.

AN ENZYMATIC FUNCTION FOR SRC PROTEIN

In the initial experiments, the src protein was detected by allowing radioactive amino acids (serving, in effect, as labels) to become incorporated into its amino acid chain during its synthesis in the cell. The resulting radiolabeled src protein was then precipitated from cell extracts with anti-src antibodies. Such characterization revealed the size of the protein and its presence in a variety of cell types, but afforded little insight into how it works. The biochemical function of src proteins remained obscure until radioactive ATP, a potential donor of phosphate to phosphoproteins, was added to complexes of nonradioactive src protein bound to antibodies. This provoked the radiolabeling of the antibody molecules and of the src protein itself, indicating that radioactive phosphate was being transferred biochemically from the ATP molecule to amino acids in these proteins. (See the illustration on page 88.) The result indicated that src protein can function as a protein kinase (an enzyme that takes a phosphate group from an ATP molecule and attaches it to one or more target proteins). In the simple reaction performed in a test tube, the target proteins were antibodies and p60^{src}. Within a living cell, many proteins might be potential targets for the src kinase activity.

This extraordinary finding raised the possibility that transformation by v-src was accomplished by the enzymatic transfer of phosphate groups to such target proteins; once phosphorylated by the src kinase, these target proteins might create the biological changes observed in src-transformed cells. This premise that kinase activity of the v-src protein is fundamental to its biological activity has been vindicated with a simple but dramatic experiment. When a single amino acid of p60$^{\text{v-src}}$ is changed within the region that normally binds ATP, the mutant v-src protein is made in normal amounts, but it has no protein kinase activity whatsoever. Now it totally lacks the capacity to transform cells.

Initially it was believed that the src protein kinase, like many other protein kinases known at the time, phosphorylates the amino acids serine and threonine, but in 1980 it was discovered that the phosphorylated residues on its target proteins are the amino acid tyrosine. This was most surprising, in part because less than 0.1 percent of the phosphorylated amino acids in cellular protein are phosphotyrosine. But it was also exciting, because it implied that oncogenic change could be caused by an unusual enzymatic activity, whose targets might be easy to identify since they bore this unusual signature. Indeed, it was soon learned that transformation by the v-src oncogene causes as much as a tenfold increase in total cellular

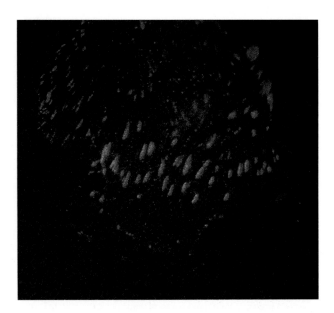

Src protein (identified with fluorescent antibodies) in RSV transformed cells is concentrated in portions of the plasma membrane (adherence plaques) that attach the cells to the surface on which they are growing.

phosphotyrosine by adding phosphate groups to 40 or more distinct cellular target proteins.

The possibility of determining which of these targets are important for cellular transformation by v-src seemed to improve when most of the v-src protein molecules within transformed cells were found to be localized to a relatively small, restricted region—the inner side of the cell membrane, especially where the membrane is attached to the surface of a culture plate. Conventional wisdom held that most of the important regulatory events in a cell, particularly control of gene expression, occurs in the nucleus, and oncogenic proteins were expected to act there. (One of the few oncogenic proteins then known, the T antigen of SV40, is indisputably located in the nucleus.) Finding src protein at the periphery of the cell was one of many surprising discoveries of the late 1970s and early 1980s that refocused attention upon cytoplasmic events in the regulation of cell growth.

The target proteins that are crucial for transformation by v-src have yet to be identified. In the meantime, however, many other proteins encoded by proto-oncogenes or otherwise implicated in the control of cell growth have been found to function, like the src proteins, as protein kinases, often specific for tyrosine residues. Furthermore, addition of phosphate groups is now known to have dramatic effects on the behavior of proteins, providing an explanation for how a single protein kinase may affect cell behavior by changing the activities of diverse proteins to which it adds phosphate groups. Protein kinases, moreover, may themselves be regulated by yet other enzymes: the activity of src protein kinases, for example, is governed by the presence or absence of

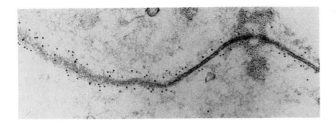

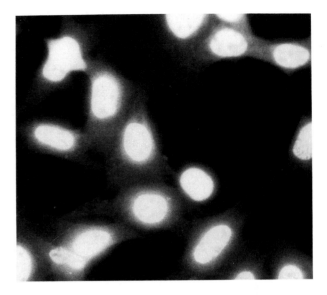

Oncogenic proteins can act in different parts of the cell. The src protein of RSV is found on the inner face of the plasma membrane (seen above in two adjacent cells, with src protein detected in the electron microscope with antibodies tagged with gold particles). The T antigen of SV40 virus is abundant in the nucleus, as shown at right with fluorescent antibodies.

phosphate groups at several positions along its amino acid chain. These phosphate groups seem to be affixed by other kinases, raising the possibility of a succession of phosphorylation events—a cascade of signals passed sequentially from one protein molecule to the next. Such regulation is lost, and the v-src kinase is persistently hyperactive, as a result of the few amino acid differences between c-src and v-src proteins. We will return to this important regulatory theme in Chapter 6.

OTHER ONCOGENIC KINASES

Protein-tyrosine kinases like the v-src protein and the related protein encoded by the viral oncogene v-abl have proved to be among the proteins most frequently implicated in experimental and human cancer. These tyrosine-specific kinases can now be recognized simply by inspection of their amino acid sequences,

which are most easily deduced from the nucleotide sequence of their genes. All the tyrosine kinases have a set of common amino acid sequences that indicate common structural features and biochemical functions. These kinases fall into two major classes. Some, like the src protein, are located entirely within the cytoplasm, although these associate with proteins integral to the cell membrane. The other class extends through the cell membrane, the leading (aminoterminal) half of the molecule protruding into the extracellular environment and the other (carboxyterminal) half remaining in the cytoplasm. Most if not all of these so-called transmembrane proteins serve as receptors for soluble extracellular factors: their external domain recognizes the presence of these factors and transmits news of the encounter to the cytoplasmic domain, which harbors the tyrosine-specific protein kinase. The enzyme responds by becoming activated and phosphorylates target proteins in the cytoplasm.

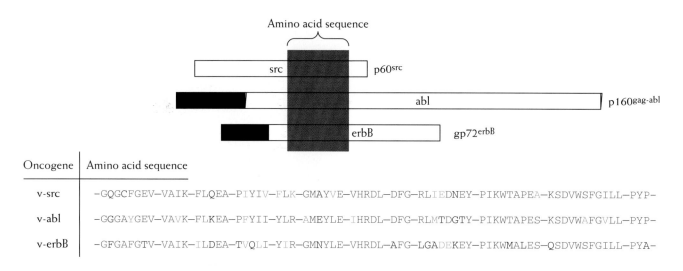

Oncogene	Amino acid sequence
v-src	–GQGCFGEV–VAIK–FLQEA–PIYIV–FLK–GMAYVE–VHRDL–DFG–RLIEDNEY–PIKWTAPEA–KSDVWSFGILL–PYP–
v-abl	–GGGAYGEV–VAVK–FLKEA–PFYII–YLR–AMEYLE–IHRDL–DFG–RLMTDGTY–PIKWTAPES–KSDVWAFGVLL–PYP–
v-erbB	–GFGAFGTV–VAIK–ILDEA–TVQLI–YIR–GMNYLE–VHRDL–AFG–LGADEKEY–PIKWMALES–QSDVWSFGILL–PYA–

Oncogenic proteins with tyrosine-specific protein kinase activity have similar amino acid sequences (shown in single letter code) that can be used to predict kinase activity in the products of newly discovered genes. Identical amino acids are shown in red, closely related ones in blue.

Some oncogenic proteins are kinases that add phosphate to serine or threonine; but because serine and threonine are so commonly phosphorylated in cells, it is extremely difficult to discern the immediate targets and effects of these transforming kinases. Nevertheless, there is accumulating evidence that serine and threonine kinases are also pivotal elements in the biochemical pathways that regulate growth.

RAS PROTEINS

In the late 1970s, methods similar to those used to identify src proteins were also vigorously applied to the characterization of ras proteins. Antisera from animals bearing v-ras-induced tumors precipitated relatively small proteins (around 190 amino acids in length and 21,000 daltons in mass, hence called p21^{ras}) from cells transformed by Harvey and Kirsten strains of murine sarcoma virus. Like the p60^{src} proteins, p21^{ras} molecules were found mainly at the cell periphery, loosely associated with the inner surface of the plasma membrane.

The ras proteins, however, are not protein kinases. Rather, the biochemical property first associated with p21^{ras} was an ability to bind guanine nucleotides, especially guanosine diphosphate (GDP) and triphosphate (GTP)—not ATP. The significance of this property became apparent over the next several years, as it was appreciated that ras proteins are related—both by amino acid sequence and by biochemical behavior—to an important class of proteins known as G (guanine-binding) proteins. These G proteins are larger than p21^{ras} proteins and also bind to GDP and GTP. Both

Structure of the ras Protein

By diffracting X rays through ordered crystals composed of a single protein, the position of virtually every atom in the protein can be determined. Powerful images emerge from such studies, inviting predictions about what the protein does, what kinds of molecules it interacts with, and how it can be affected by mutations or inhibited by drugs. So far, structures have been determined for only a few proteins implicated in growth control, among them are growth hormone and the external portion of its receptor, the protein kinase regulated by cyclic AMP, two transcription factors that interact with DNA, and p21^{ras} (shown here).

A notable feature of the ras protein is the binding site for GTP; the nucleotide is in contact with the amino acid residues (at positions 12, 13, 59, and 61) that are commonly mutated in oncogenic forms of the protein. It makes sense that these positions are close to the bound nucleotide, since the oncogenic forms are unable to convert GTP to GDP, implying a defect in the active site for GTP breakdown. Substitution of GTP for GDP (and vice versa) subtly alters the position of the effector loop, composed of amino acid residues 33 to 40. Ras mutants with changes in these amino acids cannot send a growth signal to the next point in the chain of command and cannot respond to GTPase activating protein (GAP). GAP is thought to turn off normal ras proteins by promoting conversion of GTP to GDP and to transmit the ras signal downstream.

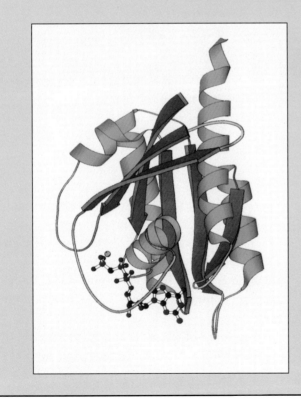

A ribbon drawing of the three-dimensional structure of p21 bound to GTP (ball-and-stick figure) as determined by X-ray crystallography. The loop at the lower left is the so-called effector loop that interacts with the GTPase activating protein. The gray ball is an associated ion of magnesium.

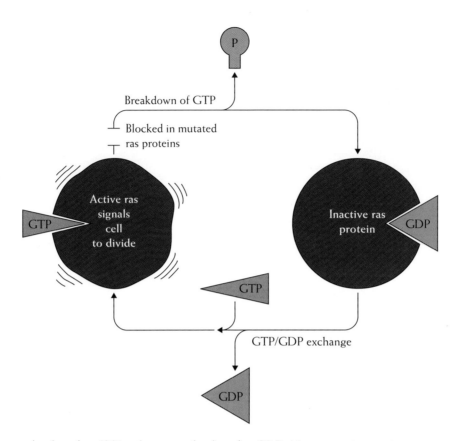

Ras proteins are active when bound to GTP and inactive when bound to GDP. Mutant proteins remain in the active state because they cannot convert GTP to GDP.

types of protein are thought to be signal-transducing: they receive a signal from an upstream component in a signaling pathway and then pass it down to the next component.

To function as signal transducers, these proteins alternate between two states in which either GDP or GTP is bound. Thus p21^{ras} is in an inactive, resting state when bound to GDP. When a stimulatory signal arrives, p21^{ras} releases its GDP and acquires a GTP molecule; with this exchange, it enters an active state in which it emits a signal to some downstream target. Shortly thereafter, p21^{ras} cleaves a phosphate group from its bound GTP molecule, reducing it to GDP, and reenters a quiescent state.

Single amino acid changes distinguish the oncogenic forms of p21^{ras} from the normal version. These changes affect one important aspect of p21^{ras} function: while oncogenic p21^{ras} forms can bind GTP and assume an active, signal-emitting state, they are unable to turn off their signal transmission by breaking down the GTP to GDP. As a result, trapped indefinitely in the active state, they inappropriately flood the cell with unremitting signals—in this case presumably growth-promoting signals. The ras switch, in effect, gets stuck in the "on" position.

This model, however, does not reveal precisely how an oncogenic form of p21^{ras} transforms a cell. What is the nature of the biochemical signal that p21 emits? What is its target? Since ras proteins are not known to have enzymatic functions except to degrade GTP to GDP, p21^{ras} is assumed to act as a regulator of yet another protein endowed with enzymatic activity, such as a protein kinase. But the identity of the proteins directly affected by activated p21^{ras} remains elusive.

NUCLEAR PROTEINS

Not all oncogenes and proto-oncogenes encode proteins found in the cytoplasm or associated with the plasma membrane. The c-myc gene is one of the first and most important to be shown to encode a nuclear protein. Recent evidence, discussed in Chapter 6, indicates that protein products of c-myc, of other myc genes, and of several other proto-oncogenes regulate transcription of a cohort of target genes in the nucleus by binding to their DNA

sequences, allowing or disallowing them to be read out in the form of messenger RNA.

Among the most important and best studied of these transcriptional regulators are the fos and jun proteins. First identified as the products of retroviral oncogenes and their cellular progenitors, fos and jun each belong to a small family of related proteins. Members of each family can combine with members of the other to create dimers (such as fos–jun complexes) with varied activities. One such dimer is the well-known transcription control factor AP-1, produced in large amounts when many kinds of cells are stimulated to enter the cell growth cycle. Unfortunately, very little is known about the target genes regulated by this class of transcription factors.

OTHER ONCOGENIC PROTEINS: GROWTH FACTORS AND RECEPTORS

Methods for characterizing the protein product of an isolated gene have advanced rapidly over the past few years; the slow unveiling of src, ras, and myc protein functions seems clumsy in retrospect. For a newly discovered gene, it is now standard practice to deduce the amino acid sequences of its protein product by determining the nucleotide sequences of DNA clones of the gene or of its messenger RNA. Antibodies that react with its protein can then be produced by immunizing rabbits or mice, using chemically synthesized or bacterially produced fragments of the protein as antigens.

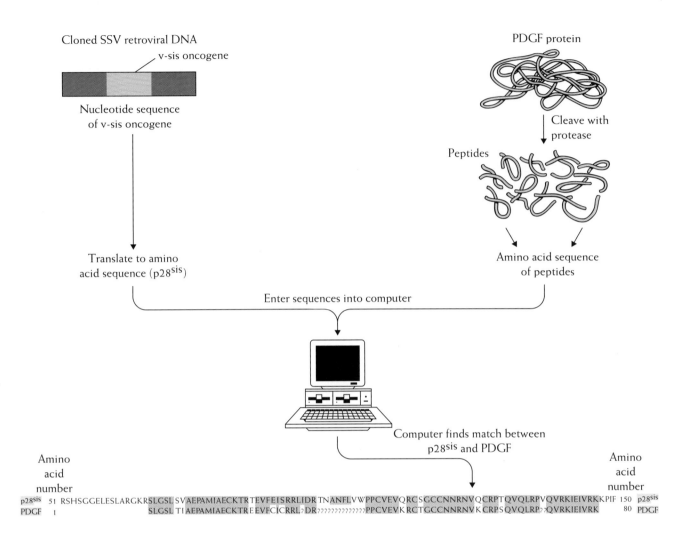

Cloned SSV retroviral DNA

v-sis oncogene

Nucleotide sequence
of v-sis oncogene

Translate to amino
acid sequence (p28^{sis})

PDGF protein

Cleave with
protease

Peptides

Amino acid sequence
of peptides

Enter sequences into computer

Computer finds match between
p28^{sis} and PDGF

Amino
acid
number

Amino
acid
number

p28^{sis} 51 RSHSGGELESLARGKRSLGSL SVAEPAMIAECKTRTEVFEISRRLIDR TNANFLVWPPCVEVQRCSGCCNNRNVQCRPTQVQLRPVQVRKIEIVRKKPIF 150 p28^{sis}
PDGF   1   SLGSL TIAEPAMIAECKTREEVFCICRRL?DR?????????????PPCVEVKRCTGCCNNRNVKCRPSQVQLRP??QVRKIEIVRK   80 PDGF

Computer-based comparisons of amino acid sequences determined by direct analysis of PDGF (right)
and by nucleotide sequencing of the v-sis oncogene revealed that the sis proto-oncogene is the gene
encoding a subunit of the growth factor PDGF.

The antisera can be used, in turn, to determine the cellular localization of the protein and to characterize its chemical modifications, enzymatic activities, and associations with other proteins. It is now often possible to predict important properties of a protein long before any direct biochemical analysis of the protein has been undertaken, by making use of the large collections of sequences of other proteins that have been stored in computerized data bases. Structural similarities with other, known proteins may predict the location of an oncogenic protein within the cell, its chemical modifications, or its enzymatic activities.

In 1983, one of the first and most striking of these similarities was found between the amino acid sequence of the protein product of a viral oncogene (the v-sis gene of simian sarcoma virus) and the sequence of a secreted growth factor, human platelet-derived growth factor (PDGF). The link indicated that the deregulated production by an oncogene of a growth-stimulatory factor could lead to cell transformation. This growth factor is usually secreted by one cell, diffuses through the intercellular space, and acts on a second cell, which senses its presence and responds by proliferating. The sis oncogene forces a tumor cell to secrete large amounts of a PDGF-like growth factor, which apparently stimulates growth of the cell that has just released it. (Other oncogenes also seem to specify secreted growth factors that act in an autostimulatory, or autocrine, fashion to force cell growth.)

This discovery also suggested that oncogenes may function by creating growth-stimu-latory signals belonging to the same signaling pathways normally exploited by growth factors like PDGF. This idea was confirmed by discoveries that the v-erbB and v-fms oncogenes are derived from genes that specify normal cellular growth-factor receptors—proteins used by the cell to detect the presence of growth factors in the extracellular space. The aberrant receptor proteins encoded by the v-erbB and v-fms oncogenes release continuous growth signals into the cell, through the agency of their tyrosine-specific protein kinase activities on the cytoplasmic face of the cell membrane. Their normal counterparts, in contrast, release such signals only after they have recognized and bound appropriate extracellular growth factors.

GENERAL FEATURES OF PROTO-ONCOGENE PRODUCTS

It is striking that proteins implicated in oncogenesis display such a diversity of locations and biochemical functions. This suggests that these proteins can meddle in cellular growth control at a large number of points. The presence of many oncoproteins outside the nucleus implies that important changes in cellular behavior can be caused by events distant from the sites where DNA is replicated and transcribed. That a remarkable number of these proteins are protein kinases stresses the importance of phosphorylation in the regulation of protein function and the control of cell prolif-

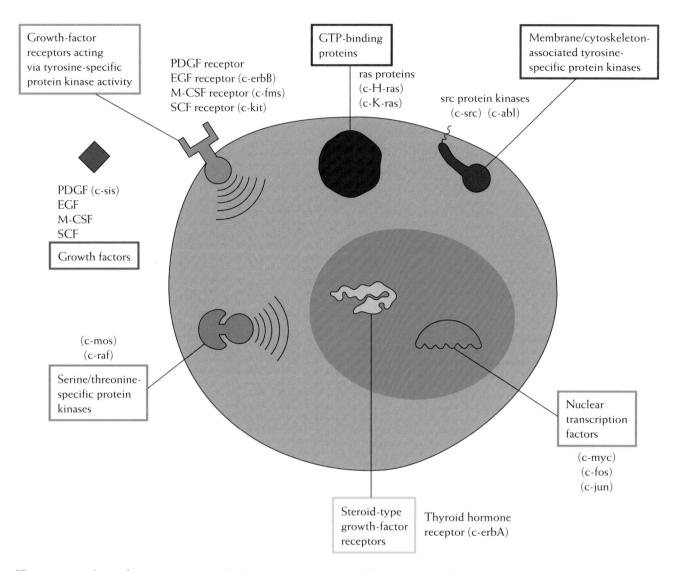

Growth-factor
receptors acting
via tyrosine-specific
protein kinase activity

PDGF receptor
EGF receptor (c-erbB)
M-CSF receptor (c-fms)
SCF receptor (c-kit)

GTP-binding
proteins

ras proteins
(c-H-ras)
(c-K-ras)

Membrane/cytoskeleton-
associated tyrosine-
specific protein kinases

src protein kinases
(c-src) (c-abl)

PDGF (c-sis)
EGF
M-CSF
SCF

Growth factors

(c-mos)
(c-raf)

Serine/threonine-
specific protein
kinases

Nuclear
transcription
factors

(c-myc)
(c-fos)
(c-jun)

Steroid-type
growth-factor
receptors

Thyroid hormone
receptor (c-erbA)

The protein products of proto-oncogenes and related genes have many different biochemical functions performed at several places inside a cell or in the extracellular space.

eration. Many of the proteins involved in cellular growth control are related to each other by sequence and function; they are encoded by members of gene families that have common evolutionary origins and may be partially redundant in their functions.

The functions normally delegated to these various proteins can be intensified or skewed by mutations that change the protein structure or produce normal proteins in abnormally large amounts. Excessive concentrations of an extracellular growth factor, unbridled catalytic activity of a mutant protein-tyrosine kinase, or inappropriately high levels of a transcription factor can each have detrimental effects upon the control of cell growth; even in the presence of a normal copy of the corresponding proto-oncogene, an oncogene may disrupt the carefully balanced molecular controls on cell proliferation to such an extent that malignant growth ensues.

Before assessing the mechanisms by which such dominant mutations derail growth control, we must consider another aspect of the problem: tumor suppressor genes, the subject of the next chapter. These genes participate in tumorigenesis when mutations eliminate or reduce their normal growth-inhibitory actions; they present a mirror image of the proto-oncogenes just described.

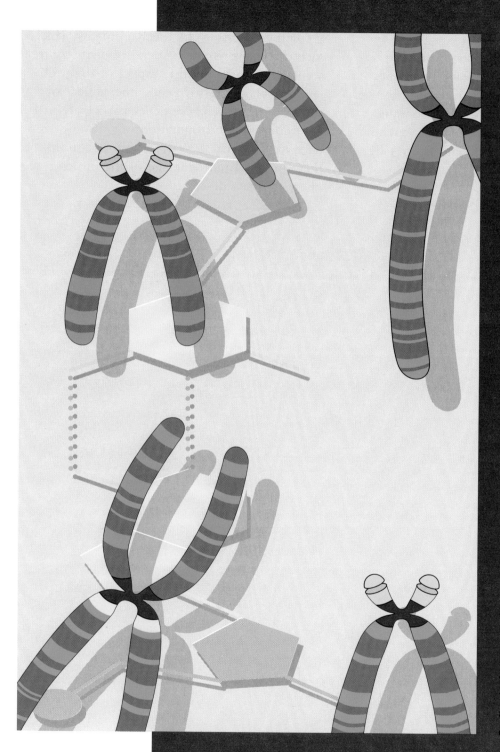

An artist's fanciful depiction of human chromosomes 3, 5, 13, 14, and 17 with the molecular structure of DNA bases in the background. Deletions of specific bands in these chromosomes (shown here in green) have been found in certain types of tumor cells. This observation suggested the presence of specific growth-inhibiting genes in the discarded chromosomal regions—genes that were eventually identified as the tumor suppressor genes described in this chapter.

THE GENETIC ELEMENTS GOVERNING CANCER: TUMOR SUPPRESSOR GENES

O ncoproteins, as we have seen, can trigger malignant cell transformation by activating the pathways that regulate cell proliferation in response to mitogens. But these well-studied proteins and the pathways in which they operate are not the sole regulators of cell growth and differentiation. An array of equally potent genes and their products suppresses cell growth.

Tissues seem to use two strategies to limit cell proliferation. The first depends upon rationing of the mitogenic signals that stimulate normal cell growth. For example, the production and release of several mitogenic growth factors, such as platelet-derived growth factor (PDGF) and fibroblast growth factor (FGF), are very tightly controlled in normal tissues. The second strategy relies upon regulators that actively suppress proliferation. These genes, called suppressor genes, tumor suppressor genes, or even anti-oncogenes, appear to be as important as proto-oncogenes in governing normal cell proliferation. Growth-suppressing genes can play an important role in the creation of tumor cells. When one of these genes is inactivated, the cell cannot curb its own proliferation, and excessive cell growth may result.

If we think of the cellular growth-regulating system as an automobile, the oncogenes can be considered the accelerator and the growth-suppressing genes the brake. Excessive cell growth can result from either a stuck accelerator (activated oncogene) or a defective brake (inactivated tumor suppressor gene).

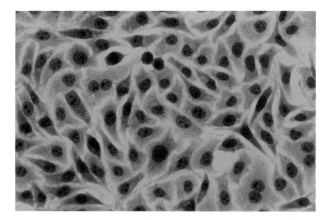

A cell population before fusion (above) and immediately after fusion (right). Note the multinucleated cells in the fused population.

DISCOVERY OF TUMOR SUPPRESSORS

The very existence of tumor suppressor genes was difficult to prove. Because they normally constrain cell proliferation, these genes are revealed only when they are lost and cells start to grow uncontrollably. This creates a quandary: the cancer biologist must study a gene whose workings only become apparent long after it has been silenced or lost. Thus, we cannot examine these genes directly but must resort to indirect experimental strategies.

Clues about the existence of the tumor suppressor genes first surfaced with a puzzling observation suggesting that, under certain circumstances, normal cells seem to dominate the behavior of aggressive cancer cells. The experiments that led to this apparent paradox used cell fusion, a technique in which neighboring cells growing at the bottom of a culture dish are fused to one another. Exposure of a cell monolayer to Sendai virus particles or to the chemical polyethylene glycol causes the outer

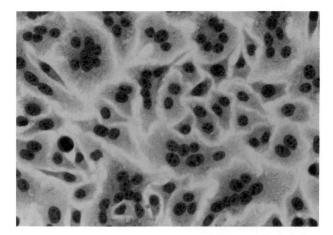

membranes of neighboring cells to fuse together. The cytoplasms of several cells unite into one large, shared cytoplasm that includes several cell nuclei. Some of these multinucleated cells die, but others grow normally and divide. In the fused cells, the chromosomes from several nuclei congregate into the single common nucleus that soon forms. In this way, the genes of the two (or more) parent cells are pooled and together determine the behavior of the hybrid cell.

In the late 1960s, researchers fused normal cells with cancer cells to study the growth traits of the resulting normal–malignant hybrids. Two outcomes were possible. The genes donated by the tumor cell parent might dominate the hybrid cells, which would then form tumors when inoculated into a suitable host animal such as a mouse. Alternatively, genes originating from the normal parent cell might dominate, in which case the descendant hybrid cells would not form tumors in a host animal. As it turned out, such hybrid cells almost always lacked the ability to form tumors in animals. The traits of the normal cells indeed dominated those of the cancer cells to which they became fused, a result that runs counter to the intuition that the genes of the virulent, malignant cancer cell would dominate those of the benign normal partner.

There was only one simple way to explain this outcome: the normal cell must have contributed some tumor-suppressing activity that imposed normal growth behavior on the hybrid cell. This mysterious activity could come, in principle, from any component of the normal cell—its cytoplasmic proteins, its protein-synthesis machinery, or its genes. The fact that descendants of the hybrid cell often remained nontumorigenic for many generations, however, pointed to a cell factor that was stably transmitted from generation to generation, thereby implicating genes in the process.

In short, normal cells seemed to carry genes that could suppress the malignant behavior of tumor cells. These genes might constrain growth in normal cells and, when inactivated, lead to the unconstrained growth of tumor cells. When such genes were introduced into tumor cells by fusion, the cancer cells reacquired an important component of the growth-regulating machinery that their ancestors discarded many cell generations earlier. Responding to this newly restored machinery, the cancer cells reverted to a normal growth pattern and no longer formed tumors. In effect, these tumor suppressor genes reimposed normal growth control on the tumor cells.

A bit more was learned about these genes by studying the chromosomes in the hybrids. When hybrid cells are initially formed through fusion, their nuclei carry two complete sets of chromosomes, one from each parent cell. This is twice as many chromosomes as a cell usually possesses. Consequently, as the hybrid cell and its descendants proceed through multiple rounds of growth and division, they often discard some of these extra chromosomes, thereby reducing their total collection to a more normal, manageable size. Sometimes the chromosomes lost from a hybrid cell originate from the normal parent cell. With the loss of these normal chromosomes comes the loss of certain genes that had previously forced the hybrid cell to grow normally. Once the hybrid cell discards these growth-normalizing chromosomes and associated genes, it reverts at once by showing traits of its malignant ancestor.

This behavior provided a useful technique for tracking the elusive tumor suppressor genes. If reversion of the nonmalignant hybrid cells to the cancerous state was found always to be accompanied by the loss of a particular chromosome, that chromosome (and not one of the 23 others) probably carried a critical suppressor gene. For example, human sarcoma cells were found to lose tumorigenicity when fused to normal fibroblasts. As these hybrids were passed in culture, they lost copies of chromosomes donated by the normal parent and occasionally reverted to cancerous behavior. In particular, the loss of normal human chromosome 11 correlated with their reversion to tumorigenicity. This indicated that the nor-

mal human chromosome 11 carries a gene (or genes) that normalizes sarcoma cell growth, thereby blocking neoplastic proliferation by the hybrid. Further, an ancestor of the sarcoma cells must have lost copies of the chromosome 11 gene during its earlier evolution from normality to malignancy.

Although these experiments gave valuable clues about the existence of these genes, a more specific description of their structure and functioning was needed.

ISOLATION OF A TUMOR SUPPRESSOR GENE

Fortunately, there are more direct ways to demonstrate that gene loss occurs during the development of tumors. Cytologists studying chromosome structure can sometimes see the loss of genetic material in a light microscope, especially when the chromosomes are prepared from cells that are in mitosis. Blue/purple staining of chromosomes in the metaphase stage brings out much of their fine structure, highlighted by arrays of dark-staining bands interspersed with light-staining regions. Such banding patterns differ from one chromosome to the next; within each chromosome, they serve to identify and demarcate specific subchromosomal regions. Each of these chromosomal bands carries a stretch of DNA long enough to encode dozens of genes.

Using a catalogue of these chromosomal bands as a reference, cytologists surveyed the chromosomes associated with the creation of cancer cells. In one well-studied case, a spe-

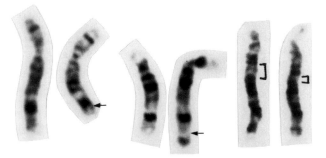

Two important, readily observed chromosomal anomalies of cancer cells. Left two pairs: A translocation in which the tip of the left chromosome of each pair has broken off and been added to the end of the right chromosome of each pair (arrows). Right pair: An interstitial deletion causes the loss of a usually visible band (compare brackets).

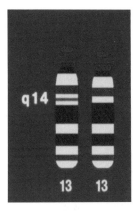

Interstitial deletion of the q14 band of chromosome 13 seen in some retinoblastomas; compare left (normal band) and right (deleted band). Microscopic observation of this deletion suggested that this region contains a critical gene, later designated Rb.

THE RETINOBLASTOMA MODEL

Retinoblastoma tumors are very rare, being seen in only one out of 20,000 children. These tumors occur early in life and are seldom seen after the age of five or six. The disease often runs in families. Many people who are cured as children will later, as adults, have offspring who are also affected. In such families, this otherwise very rare cancer may affect half the offspring, pointing to the involvement of a gene passed from parent to child that confers susceptibility. Children suffering from this familial form of retinoblastoma usually have multiple tumor foci growing in both eyes.

A second type of retinoblastoma, the sporadic form, is seen in children whose parents have no history of the disease. Once cured, these patients, as adults, will not pass the disease to the next generation. Consequently spo-

cific chromosomal aberration was seen in the cells of children suffering from retinoblastoma (a tumor of embryonic cells that develop into the retina). One band (labeled q14) situated on the long arm of chromosome 13 was occasionally missing. Such a small internal, or interstitial, deletion suggests that one or more genes lying within this chromosomal region has been discarded. It was speculated that a critical step in formation of this tumor is the loss of a specific gene (termed Rb for retinoblastoma) whose DNA is nestled somewhere in this small chromosomal region. Since this gene loss seemed to correlate with tumor formation, it appeared that the Rb gene constrains growth in normal retinal precursor cells. Thus, the Rb gene became the first tumor suppressor gene to be identified and associated with a discrete chromosomal site.

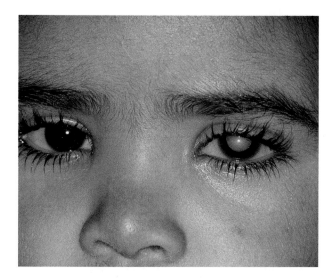

An advanced retinoblastoma in a young child.

radic retinoblastoma affects only one generation, and the affected children have only one
tumor focus, in a single eye.

A simple genetic model, originally proposed by Alfred Knudson in 1971, explains the
origins of retinoblastoma and the connection
between these two different forms of the disease. Knudson studied the timing of retinoblastoma appearance in children from cancer-prone
families and in children with the sporadic form
of the disease. Mathematical analysis convinced
him that two distinct genetic alterations are
required to create retinoblastoma tumors.

Knudson's model, subsequently vindicated,
had great impact on the study of the genetics
of human cancer. In its simplest form, the

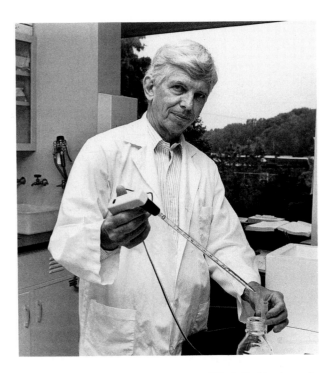

Alfred G. Knudson, Jr.

model states that children with sporadic retinoblastoma are genetically normal at the moment
of conception, but during their embryonic development two somatic mutations occur in a
cell lineage leading to the photoreceptors in
the retina: the rods and cones. The resulting
doubly mutated cell then proliferates into an
eye tumor.

In familial retinoblastoma, the fertilized egg
(zygote) already carries a mutant gene, acquired from sperm or egg, so all the cells descended from this zygote (that is, all the cells
in the body) carry this mutation, including the
cells in the developing retina. These cells now
must sustain only a single somatic mutation to
reach the doubly mutated configuration required for tumor formation. In effect, each of
the retinal cells is already primed for tumorigenesis and needs only a single event to push
it over the edge into the malignant state.

By 1983, it was clear that the two mutated
genes in Knudson's model were the two copies
of the Rb gene, first identified through microscopic examination of chromosomes. Like almost all other human genes, the Rb gene exists in duplicate in each cell; in this case each
copy is found on one of the paired chromosomes 13. Moreover, these mutations inactivate
both Rb gene copies, leaving the retinal cell
without any intact Rb gene and unleashing
cancerous growth. (In contrast, the mutations
that turn the proto-oncogenes into oncogenes
do so by activating only one copy of the
gene.)

Why does the formation of retinal tumor
cells require the loss of *both* Rb gene copies? In
mammalian cells, the presence of two copies of
most genes provides redundant function—a

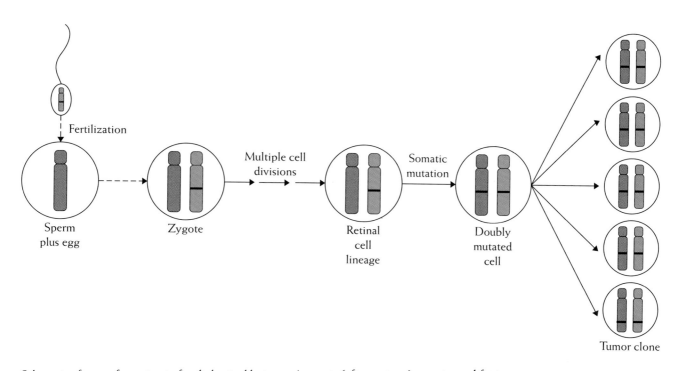

Schematic of tumor formation in familial retinoblastoma. A gamete (often a sperm) carrying a defective Rb gene forms a zygote that is heterozygous at the Rb locus (one good and one mutant gene copy). If a cell in the retinal lineage later loses the remaining good Rb gene copy to somatic mutation, the doubly mutated cell that results proliferates into a tumor.

safety backup. When a single copy of any gene pair is lost, the surviving copy can usually maintain normal cell function. Thus a single normal Rb gene copy is powerful enough to hold back unconstrained cell growth, and the retinal cells grow normally. Only when both gene copies are lost or inactivated do the cells grow uncontrollably. In children with only a single intact Rb gene copy, all cells of the developing embryo grow normally. Late in gestation, however, during the development of the eye and its retina, any retinal cell may, through random accident, lose its one surviving normal copy of the Rb gene, resulting in

excessive growth. Such accidents may occur spontaneously once in a million cell divisions, and the number of retinal cells in each eye is so large that several cells usually suffer this fate. It is estimated that 95 percent of children who are hemizygous at their Rb locus (that is, have only one normal Rb gene copy in all their cells) will develop retinal tumors.

Since loss of function in a gene is not uncommon over the millions of cell divisions that occur during embryologic development of the retina, why is retinoblastoma not seen frequently in genetically normal children? Children who have inherited two intact copies of the Rb gene may well lose one copy in several retinal cells during their embryological development, but the second copy remains as a backup in these cells. The chance of losing *both* Rb copies in the same cell is exceedingly small. Nonetheless, on very rare occasions (about one in 30,000 births), a retinoblastoma tumor will appear in a child who started out with two normal Rb genes but lost both of them in some retinal cell. This accounts for the sporadic form of the disease.

CHROMOSOME SHUFFLING

Retinoblastoma is only one of several tumors that appear to arise through loss or inactivation of critical genes regulating cell growth. Wilms' tumor of the kidney, for example, is a more common cancer whose origins have been traced to loss of a critical growth-regulating gene, termed WT-1, located on chromosome 11. Despite the manner in which the Rb and WT-1 genes were identified, the presence of most growth-suppressing genes cannot be ascertained through microscopic examination of tumor cell chromosomes. Such examination of chromosome structure yields only a view of gross, large-scale changes in DNA involving millions of base pairs. Subtle changes in nucleotide sequence involving one or a few base pairs of DNA can also knock out suppressor gene function and yet have no effect on the overall anatomy of the chromosome and its appearance in the microscope.

This limitation has forced geneticists to seek alternative strategies for uncovering tumor suppressor genes. The most fruitful of these was inspired by studying the details of the specific steps leading to the formation of retinoblastomas. Recall that Rb gene inactivation occurs in two discrete steps: the loss of one gene copy (which may occur in an ancestral cell) and the loss of the second surviving copy (which may occur many cell generations later). This second copy can be eliminated in tumor cells through a number of different genetic mechanisms. The simplest seems to involve repeating the earlier event that knocked out the first gene copy. A rare accident in DNA replication like that which created the first deletion or point mutation could occur again to inactivate the second copy.

Another, even more effective genetic mechanism occurs much more frequently. Entire regions of chromosomes may be shuffled as part of normal chromosome recombination

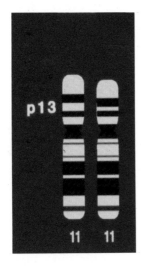

An interstitial deletion in the p13 band of chromosome 11 led to discovery of the WT-1 gene.

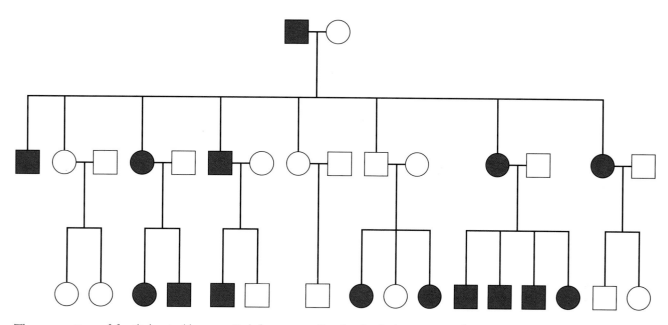

Three generations of familial retinoblastoma. Red denotes an affected individual; a square indicates a male, a circle a female.

mechanisms that result in the exchange of large domains between paired chromosomes. In effect, the paired chromosomes line up and swap equivalent segments, leaving each with a full set of genes. Such exchanges can cause one chromosomal arm to be lost and replaced by a duplicated copy of the complementary arm donated by the paired chromosome.

Such chromosome shuffling occurs during the creation of most retinoblastomas. First a

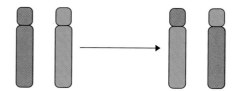

A simple schematic of chromosomal recombination.

cell loses one of its Rb genes, so that one of its chromosomes 13 carries a defective Rb gene while the other carries an intact, functional version. Then the chromosomal arm carrying the intact Rb gene copy may be replaced by a duplicated copy of the arm from the other chromosome carrying the defective gene copy.

The effect on the overall genetic makeup of the cell is minimal because the duplicated information replaces in very large part the information that was lost. But the consequences for cellular growth control can be devastating, because the cell has now lost its surviving Rb gene copy. Such loss followed by duplication is termed loss of heterozygosity. Heterozygosity refers to the unequal genetic content of two copies of a gene, in this case the two initially nonequivalent versions of the Rb gene.

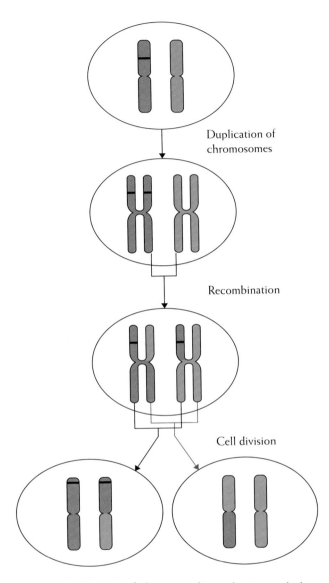

Duplication of
chromosomes

Recombination

Cell division

A schematic of chromosomal recombination, which is frequently responsible for elimination of the intact gene copy in a heterozygous cell with one inactive Rb (or other tumor suppressor) gene. Exchange of chromosomal segments occurring during mitosis leaves both daughter cells homozygous at the tumor suppressor locus, one with two defective versions of the gene (−) and the other fully wild type (normal).

Following loss and duplication, a cell becomes homozygous at its Rb locus: it has two identical (albeit defective) versions of the gene.

Because humans are genetically heterogeneous, many of the paired versions of our genes differ from one another at least subtly. Thus, heterozygosity is a normal condition at many sites throughout our genomes. This is most obvious in genes that specify visible traits such as eye color, in which one of the versions (alleles) of an eye color gene may encode a brown iris and the other a blue one. More often, heterozygosity is manifested as subtle differences in the structure of a protein encoded by the cell's two gene copies or simply as differences in the nucleotide sequences of the two copies. Even DNA sequences that fall between genes, rather than within a single gene, may differ subtly when their two copies are compared.

These differences in DNA sequence are present throughout the human genome and can often be detected through the use of specific DNA probes, each of which recognizes a distinct region of the human genome. In this way, an experimenter can analyze the DNA from a person's normal cells and compare it with DNA extracted from tumor cells in the same individual. On occasion, the analysis will show heterozygosity (dissimilar copies) of a DNA region in the normal DNA but homozygosity (identical copies) in the tumor DNA. This result is exactly what would be expected for the DNA of a tumor suppressor gene that has lost its second, intact allele. In fact, the chances are small that the probe is recognizing the DNA of the tumor suppressor gene itself. Rather, the probe is likely to be detecting a nearby sequence on the chromosome, thereby revealing a chromosomal swap involving a very large region that includes the suppressor gene, the sequences recognized by the probe, and many other neighboring but unrelated sequences. The loss of heterozygosity in this chromosomal region, observed repeatedly in a number of tumors, suggests the existence of a tumor suppressor gene whose second, still in-

tact gene copy is being eliminated repeatedly during the course of tumor formation.

A DNA probe analysis of several dozen colon carcinomas, for example, uncovered repeated loss of heterozygosity on the long arm of chromosome 18. This result indicated that both copies of a gene located somewhere on this chromosomal arm were eliminated during the process that leads to a colon tumor. On the basis of this preliminary evidence, molecular geneticists conducted a detailed survey of this chromosomal arm, ultimately focusing on a single gene. This gene, called DCC (for "deleted in colon carcinoma"), was isolated by molecular cloning, and more than 70 percent of advanced colon tumors indeed appear to have lost both functional DCC gene copies.

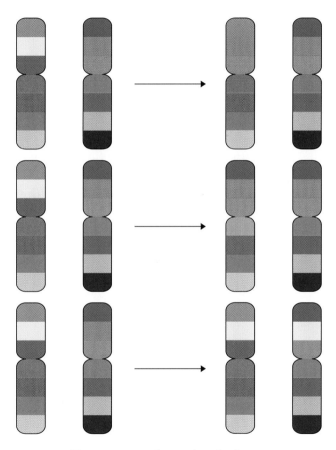

Chromosomes in three independently arising tumors: note that the same region (second band from the top) is reduced to homozygosity (represented by identical colors) in all three.

THE P53 GENE AND ITS PRODUCT

Many of the tumor suppressor genes uncovered by chromosomal mapping or isolated through molecular cloning behave very much like the Rb gene: both copies must be inactivated before a cell will begin to grow uncontrollably. A defective copy inherited in the germ line creates a familial susceptibility, because many cells in the organ affected will lose their surviving gene copies. Thus, defective inherited versions of the WT-1 gene result in Wilms' tumor, while defective versions of the NF-1 gene lead to neurofibromatosis.

One suppressor gene does not fit easily into this model: p53, by current accounts the most frequently mutated gene in human tumors. The p53 gene acts to limit cell growth,

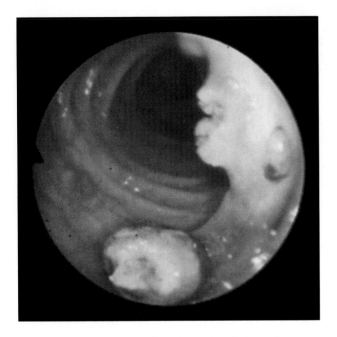

Endoscopic view of a colon polyp. Polyps often result from defects in the APC suppressor gene.

nizes and binds to a specific sequence of DNA bases that is thought to be part of the control region of certain genes, and it can stimulate the activities of RNA polymerase, the central enzyme that drives gene expression by making messenger RNA.

The p53 protein exists normally as a tetramer or perhaps a higher order aggregate. This means that four or more identical copies of the p53 protein assemble to constitute the active form of the molecule. This molecular architecture confers a peculiar liability. If any one of the four subunits is defective—suffering an amino acid replacement or some other minor structural defect, for instance—it may, like the bad apple in a barrel, compromise the function of the remaining three subunits. When a cell has one good (wild type) and one defective allele of p53, most of its p53 function may be compromised because most of the p53 tetramers will have at least one bad subunit. All the possible ways the good (+) and bad (−) p53 copies can aggregate are shown below.

Only one (++++) of these 16 tetramers, all of which are equally likely to be formed in a genetically heterozygous (+, −) cell, is fully functional. The others may be partially or even totally defective if a single p53 subunit suffices to knock out the function of a whole tetramer. This means that a single defective p53 gene

but the genetic mechanisms that involve it in cancer are very different from those that affect the Rb, WT-1, NF-1, and DCC genes.

The p53 protein (named for its molecular weight of 53,000) was discovered long before the gene that specifies its structure. Like Rb and WT-1, it is a nuclear protein apparently involved in regulating the expression of a suite of cellular genes. How it does this is not completely clear, but we do know that it recog-

			+ + + +			
	− + + +	+ − + +		+ + − +	+ + + −	
− − + +	− + − +	− + + −		+ − − +	+ − + −	+ + − −
	+ − − −	− + − −		− − + −	− − − +	
			− − − −			

Tumor Suppressor Genes Isolated by Gene Cloning		
CHROMOSOMAL LOCATION	**NAME OF GENE**	**DISEASE**
5q21	APC	Familial polyposis
11p13	WT-1	Wilms' tumor
13q14	Rb	Retinoblastoma, osteosarcoma
17p12-13	p53	Li-Fraumeni syndrome, many tumor types
17q11	NF-1	Von Recklinghausen neurofibromatosis
18q21	DCC	Colon carcinoma

copy may severely affect p53 function in the cell as a whole, creating downstream effects on cell behavior. In the other tumor suppressor genes, whose protein products all act as single, free molecules, there is little effect on cell behavior when one of their two copies is lost. While loss of half a gene's function seems tolerable for the cell, loss of 15/16 (as occurs with p53) apparently is not.

Many tumor cells have one good and one defective p53 gene copy. But unlike the mutations that affect most other suppressor genes, such as Rb—which usually knock out the gene function completely, leaving a dead allele that makes no protein whatsoever—the p53 mutations are almost invariably subtle changes: point mutations that cause amino acid replacements in the protein. The resulting p53 protein is in large part functionally inactive but is still able to trap normal p53 molecules in the tetrameric complexes, where they are unable to function properly. Tumor cells often discard their single remaining wild type (+) allele, become totally bereft of proper p53 function, and apparently grow even more aggressively.

SUPPRESSOR PROTEINS: A CHAIN OF COMMAND

Discovering the suppressor genes by using various experimental techniques is an exciting, challenging, and undeniably necessary part of understanding cancer. But the real problem is to figure out how these genes and their encoded proteins work. How do they retard cell growth, and what makes them do so? Here is one simple model.

Why Is the p53 Gene Involved in So Many Cancers?

p53 genes are frequently mutated in colon, lung, breast, esophageal, liver, and brain tumors, as well as in leukemia. Here are the factors that make it such a common participant in carcinogenesis:

1. Point mutations create onco-genic alleles of p53; such mutations occur with great frequency.

2. Point mutations occurring at any of more than 100 sites scattered throughout the middle of the p53 gene succeed in creating cancer-causing alleles of p53. This is a large target size compared with the half-dozen sites at which point mutations succeed in making activated ras oncogenes. (Mutations elsewhere in the ras gene do not cause cancer because they do not make oncogenic versions of this gene.)

3. A single mutant p53 gene copy is enough to perturb cell growth.

4. p53 seems to be an important growth regulator in a wide variety of cell types.

Each suppressor gene encodes a signal-transducing protein that relays growth-inhibiting messages from one part of the cell to another. Such proteins receive growth-suppressing signals from higher up in a signaling cascade and pass them on further down to a subordinate, responder protein. When a suppressor protein is eliminated because of mutation of its gene copies, a vital link in the signaling chain of command is lost, and growth-inhibitory signals normally transmitted through this pathway will no longer reach their intended destination.

The earlier analogy with the brake pedal of a car is useful here. A brake pedal does not decide to slow down or stop the car; it only transduces a signal, in this case by acquiring a command from the driver and passing it on to the master brake cylinder, which in turn sends signals to the brake shoes via a series of hydraulic lines. This mechanical signaling cascade involves a number of signal-transducing intermediaries: the brake pedal, the master cylinder, the hydraulic lines, the local cylinders at each wheel, and the brake shoes they activate. A defect in any one of these elements can compromise the braking process—seriously, if it is near the top of the cascade; less seriously, if it is near the bottom and affects only one of four brakes.

This type of scenario probably applies to the operation of tumor suppressor genes and to the proteins that they encode. To prove this model, it is necessary to identify both the initial provoking stimulus—the cellular equivalent of the driver—and the final responding target—the cellular brake shoe that slows or shuts down cell proliferation.

WHAT INITIATES THE BRAKING PROCESS IN THE CELL?

Each cell in a tissue is constantly bombarded with both growth-stimulating and growth-inhibiting signals that come from neighboring cells. The cell's surface receptors receive these signals and pass them on to internal computational machinery, which processes all the signals as it establishes whether or not the cell should grow.

What happens if the cellular apparatus for receiving and processing growth-inhibiting signals—this computational machinery—is ren-

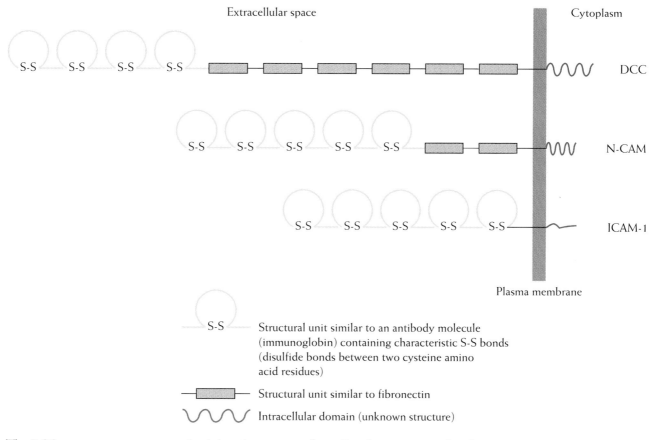

The DCC tumor suppressor protein (top) has the structure of a cell surface receptor with a large extracellular domain (left), a transmembrane domain, and an intracellular domain (right). Its structure is reminiscent of several receptors used for cell adhesion (N-CAM, middle; ICAM, bottom) with immuno-globulin-like domains (similar to those seen in antibody molecules) and fibronectin-like domains (similar to a component of the extracellular matrix).

dered defective through loss of a critical component such as a tumor suppressor protein? The cell will become unable to process these signals and so will be unresponsive, even oblivious, to them. Its growth, still urged on by growth-stimulating external signals, will no longer be held back by the signals that usually tell it not to grow.

The protein product of the DCC suppressor gene provides a good illustration of this process. The DCC protein has the structure of a cell surface receptor, indicating that it detects and receives a signal originating in the extracellular space and then relays it to the cell interior. The extracellular part of the DCC receptor appears to recognize and bind some unidentified component of the extracellular matrix—the scaffolding that holds cells together in a tissue. Contact with this matrix component seems to represent a signal that tells a normal colon cell to stop growing. If colon tumor cells lose this receptor and become insensitive to contact with the matrix component, they will continue to proliferate even when surrounded by signals telling them to stop.

WHAT ARE THE TARGETS OF GROWTH SUPPRESSION?

Inherited defective versions of the NF-1 gene, which lead to neurofibromatosis, are associated with the workings of another suppressor protein. Neurofibromatosis, erroneously termed "elephant man's disease," involves accessory cells of the nervous system, often the Schwann cells that cover and insulate nerve fibers. The

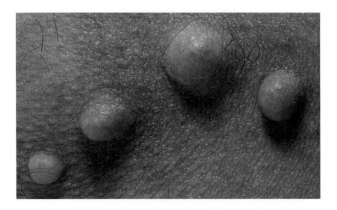

The skin of a neurofibromatosis patient displays characteristic benign tumors.

NF-1 protein functions in the cytoplasm of the cell and interacts directly with the proteins of the ras proto-oncogenes (see Chapter 4).

It is still not clear how the NF-1 protein works, but one model hypothesizes that it acts as a damper to reduce or inactivate the flow of growth-stimulating signals emitted by the ras proteins. Accordingly, cells having defective NF-1 genes and proteins may receive excess growth-stimulating signals, causing them to proliferate inappropriately. The ability of NF-1 to act as a brake may flow directly from its ability to moderate ras function. This could lead to the benign growths found in individuals with neurofibromatosis. Missing from the picture, however, is an explanation of what controls the NF-1 protein itself.

The much-discussed Rb protein is thought to bind directly to two other nuclear transcription factors that are known or suspected to promote the expression of cellular genes involved in cell growth. One of these proteins, encoded by the myc proto-oncogene, clearly plays a critical role in orchestrating cell growth through its ability to turn on other cellular genes. Does the Rb protein bind to the myc protein, trapping it and blocking it from moving around the nucleus to activate these other genes? As with NF-1, the Rb protein may brake growth by moderating the activities of growth-inducing proteins.

Although plausible and possibly correct, this model does not address the nature of the signals that regulate the activity of the Rb protein itself—the upstream signals that tell the Rb protein whether or not to brake cell growth (by sequestering transcription factors like myc). One clue comes from the phosphorylation of the Rb protein during certain parts of the cell cycle. In the amino acid sequence of the Rb protein are 10 to 12 serine and threonine amino acid residues to which phosphate groups become attached as the cell prepares for DNA synthesis. Once modified by multiple attached phosphate groups, the Rb protein

appears to lose its ability to bind to other cellular proteins, such as the transcription factors. Of course, this only pushes the question one step further: What controls the phosphorylation of Rb? We still don't know.

The Rb product is expressed in almost all types of cells throughout the body, suggesting that they must use this protein to constrain their own growth. This leads to the most puzzling, still unanswered, question concerning the Rb gene and protein: If this protein is used so widely for growth control, why does its loss lead most specifically to a tumor of the developing retina?

It turns out that Rb gene inactivation plays a role in far more than the eye tumors in which it was first discovered. Children carrying a defective Rb gene in all their cells run a several hundredfold increased risk of bone cancer (osteosarcoma) as teenagers. And one type of lung tumor frequently developed by cigarette smokers—small-cell lung carcinoma—almost invariably lacks functional Rb gene copies; in these tumors, the gene losses seem to derive largely from somatic mutations occurring because of the heavy onslaught of carcinogens in tobacco smoke. All these tumors, taken together, still represent only a small fraction of the tissues in which the Rb gene is expressed.

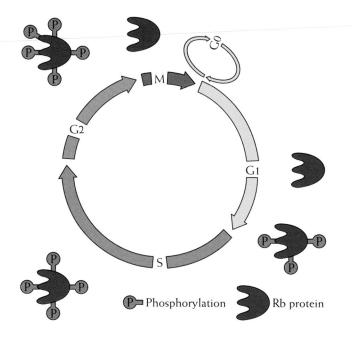

P = Phosphorylation   Rb protein

The retinoblastoma gene product, pRB, is phosphorylated at multiple sites as the cell passes into the late G1 phase and remains so until emergence from mitosis (M), at which time the phosphate groups are stripped off. Accumulating evidence suggests that pRB loses its ability to stop cell growth once it becomes phosphorylated.

Viral Oncoproteins and Suppressor Proteins

The discovery and characterization of tumor suppressor genes like p53 and Rb have solved, at least in part, a long-standing puzzle in an apparently unrelated area of cancer biology concerning DNA tumor viruses and the mechanisms they use to transform infected cells. Recall that there are two types of tumor viruses: the RNA tumor viruses, which are all members of the retrovirus class; and the DNA tumor viruses, which include polyoma virus, simian virus 40, papillomaviruses, adenoviruses, and herpesviruses.

Rapidly tumorigenic retroviruses use a straightforward mechanism to transform cells. At some time in the past, each of these viruses has picked up and activated a cellular proto-oncogene from a host cell; thereafter, each uses the activated oncogene to transform cells that it infects. This scheme works well because these viruses exploit and subvert genes and proteins that normally function as components of the cell's signaling circuitry. Consequently, it is easy for each of these retroviruses to plug its oncoprotein into the preexisting signaling circuits of the cell, thereby deregulating them.

But how do DNA tumor viruses manage this? Their oncogenes and encoded proteins are foreign to the cell, with no obvious relation to known cellular genes, so it is less clear how their viral proteins can plug into and perturb the cell's signaling circuitry.

One solution to the problem of cell transformation developed by these DNA tumor viruses is beautiful and simple. They transform cells by making viral oncoproteins that bind to, and apparently sequester, the suppressor proteins of infected cells. By tying up the cell's supply of critical suppressor proteins, these viruses mimic the state seen in spontaneous human tumor cells that have lost their suppressor proteins because the genes making them have been knocked out.

This elegant solution has been used repeatedly by a diverse group of DNA viruses. The human adenovirus E1A oncoprotein, the SV40

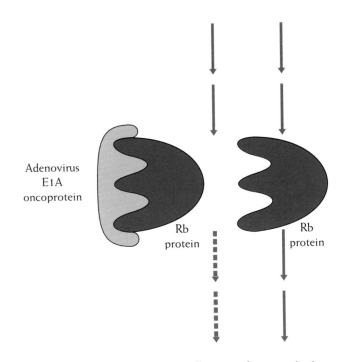

The Rb protein is normally part of a cascade that transmits growth-inhibiting signals (right). When adenovirus transforms a cell, its E1A oncoprotein binds the Rb protein (left), pulling it out of the cascade and thereby disrupting transmission of the tumor-suppressing signals (center).

large-T oncoprotein, and the E7 oncoprotein of human papillomavirus (HPV) bind to the Rb proteins of the cells they infect. HPV is strongly implicated in triggering cervical carcinoma; HPV strains whose E7 oncoprotein binds the Rb proteins only loosely are weakly carcinogenic, those that bind the Rb protein tightly are potently carcinogenic.

In all these cases, viral oncoproteins are thought to sequester the host cell's entire complement of functional Rb protein, thereby pulling it out of the regulatory circuitry. The circuitry is then crippled because it lacks a vital component, and the cell, now liberated from Rb-enforced growth suppression, can begin to grow without constraint. These three types of DNA tumor viruses also dispatch oncoproteins to cripple the p53 function of the infected host cell: adenovirus using its E1B oncoprotein, SV40 using its large-T oncoprotein, and HPV using its E6 oncoprotein. Because these viruses all target Rb and p53 proteins, it seems clear that both proteins must be inactivated if the virus-infected cells are to become transformed. Thus, Rb and p53 must serve different functions in the cell.

The strategy used by the HPV E6 protein is particularly devious: instead of binding and sequestering the p53 protein, E6 attaches itself to p53 and then attracts a host-cell protease usually used to break down protein molecules that have outlived their usefulness. Through this ruse, E6 causes p53 to be rapidly digested by the protease; indeed, almost as soon as new p53 molecules are made they are killed off. This deprives the cell of the substantial amounts of active p53 protein that it needs to shut down its own growth.

As we learn more about tumor suppressor genes, it becomes increasingly apparent that their roles in the genesis of cancer are as important as those of the more notorious, well-studied oncogenes. In certain types of tumors, inactivation of suppressor genes may be even more important than oncogene activation.

Most illustrative may be the case of colon carcinoma, which will be discussed in Chapter 7. In colon cancer cells, ras oncogene activation is found together with inactivation of the DCC and p53 tumor suppressor genes. Both types of change seem to work together to create malignant growth. Oncogene activation provides the cell with a strong, unrelenting impetus to grow; inactivation of tumor suppressor genes releases the cell from constraints that normally hinder growth. We seem to be well on our way to understanding the entire process of malignant growth deregulation in terms of these master controllers of cellular behavior.

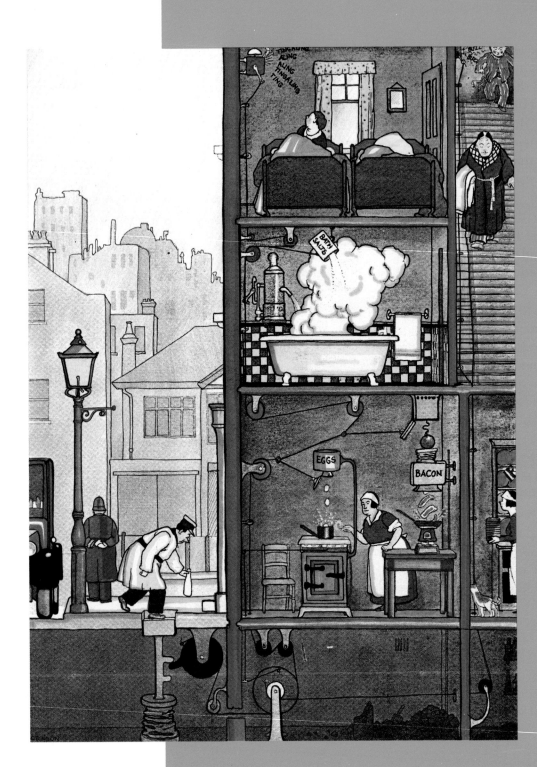

A metaphor for cell signaling, with the milkman as an external stimulating factor in the control of internal events.

6

DISTORTION OF GROWTH CONTROL IN CANCER CELLS

O ur newly acquired ability to identify the mutant genes in cancer cells and to analyze their associated mutations is a great advance in oncology. But a satisfying picture of the events that lead to cancer will ultimately require an understanding of physiological consequences: Why do such mutations lead to cancer? What are the normal functions of the genes they affect? How do cancer-promoting mutations alter those functions?

To answer these questions, we must first focus on how a normal cell receives and processes the signals from its environment that promote or inhibit its growth. These signals are keys to understanding the processes in the cell that ultimately determine its fate,

After years of working in a makeshift laboratory in Turin, Italy, during World War II, Rita Levi-Montalcini observed in 1950 in St. Louis, Missouri, that mouse sarcoma cells, implanted into developing chicken embryos, could dramatically stimulate the outgrowth of nerve fibers toward the engrafted tumors. She speculated that the growth stimulant could also circulate freely in the embryonic bloodstream after release from the cancer cells. While attempting to purify this nerve growth factor (NGF) from an alternative source—normal salivary glands—her coworker, Stanley Cohen, uncovered another strange phenomenon: his extracts could hasten the opening of the eyelids of newborn mice. In time, he ascertained that the opening was due not to NGF but to epidermal growth factor (EGF). We now recognize that NGF provokes the differentiation rather than the growth of nerve cells, whereas EGF (and its receptor) regulates the growth of many kinds of normal and cancerous cells of epithelial origin. Levi-Montalcini and Cohen shared a Nobel Prize in 1986.

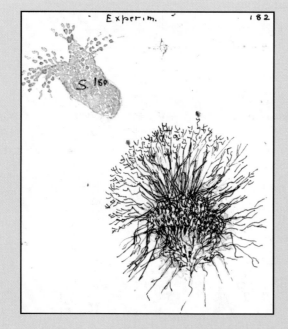

Hand drawings by Rita Levi-Montalcini of neural fibers growing out of an early chicken embryo (lower right) under the influence of nerve growth factor (NGF) produced by sarcoma cells (upper left).

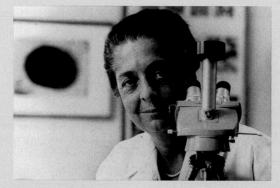

Rita Levi-Montalcini.

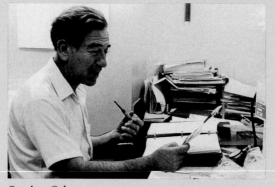

Stanley Cohen.

since a normal cell within a tissue grows, differentiates, or dies in response to external signals. This dependence for instructions on other cells, both nearby and in other parts of the body, contrasts with the autonomous behavior of a cancer cell, which is governed by its own internally generated signals. Normal cells will grow only if stimulated to do so by growth factors; cancer cells show an acquired independence from externally supplied mitogenic factors and, at the same time, may no longer respond to external growth-inhibitory signals.

Understanding how oncogenes confer growth factor autonomy will occupy the bulk of this chapter, providing a clear link between the biochemistry of growth factors and oncoproteins and the unusual biology of cancer cells. Far less is known about the biochemistry of growth suppression, which we will address briefly at the end of the chapter in the context of the loss of tumor suppressor genes. Initially we will examine how a normal cell's growth-promoting circuitry is regulated: through growth factor production; receptor function; cytoplasmic signal processing; and gene responses in the nucleus.

leave G0 and reenter the active growth cycle. The presence or absence of GFs is thus the basic element that determines whether or not a cell will grow.

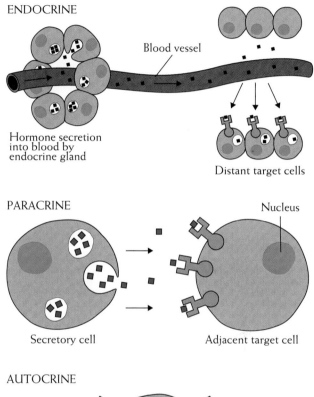

The three patterns of extracellular signaling in animals.

EXTRACELLULAR GROWTH FACTORS

In the absence of growth factors (GFs), a normal cell will exit from its growth cycle; enter the resting or quiescent state known as G0; and remain there for days, weeks, or even years. When GFs are supplied, the cell will

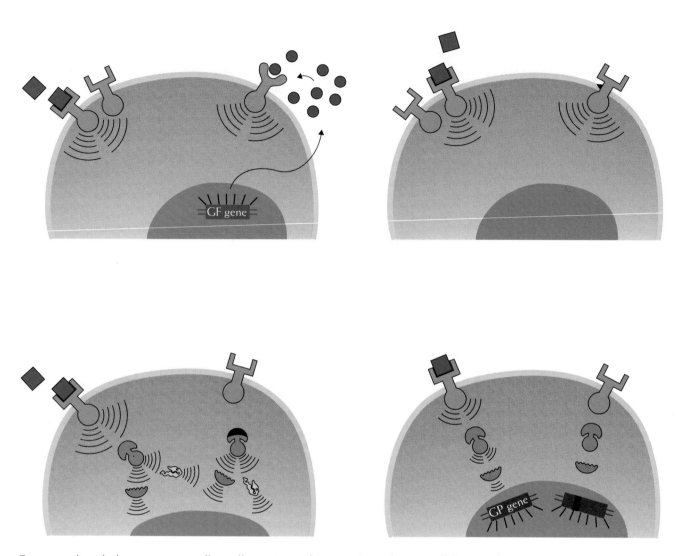

Four ways by which oncogenes can allow cells to grow without stimulation by extracellular growth factors. Top left: A normal cell requires extracellular GFs to activate its GF receptors (left); a cancer cell often makes and secretes GFs that stimulate its own growth (autocrine stimulation, right). Top right: Normal GF receptors require binding of GF to trigger signal release (left); aberrant (or overexpressed) receptors release signals into cells even without GF binding (right). Lower left: GF-activated receptors normally activate a cascade of signal transducers in the cytoplasm (left); in cancer cells, abnormal transducers in such a cascade may release growth-stimulating signals even without prompting by a GF-activated receptor (right). Lower right: In normal cells, the activation of proteins that regulate transcription of growth-promoting (GP) genes requires stimulation by cytoplasmic instructions originating with GF-activated receptors (left); in cancer cells, aberrant (or overexpressed) regulators of transcription may exist without prior stimulation by cytoplasmic receptors (right).

The specific effects upon cell growth of particular extracellular factors are intimately linked to how the factors are produced: continuously, or episodically in response to need; at one site, or many; in a fashion that allows the factors to migrate to distant cells, or one that restricts their action to adjacent cells. Many familiar factors—such as growth hormones, insulin, and glucocorticoid hormones—are produced by cells in distant organs (respectively, the pituitary gland, the islet cells of the pancreas, and the adrenal cortex) and delivered throughout the body by the bloodstream; this is termed the endocrine mode of action. Other factors act mainly or exclusively in a restricted region, either upon cells in the immediate vicinity of the factor-producing cells (the paracrine mode of action) or upon the factor-producing cells themselves (autocrine signaling). Short-distance signaling is especially important during embryonic development—when similar cells located in different places in the embryo are directed by their immediate surroundings to form different types of tissues—and during certain episodes of adult life, such as when tissue injuries are repaired or an immune response to foreign substances is mounted.

PDGF AND AUTOCRINE SIGNALING

As an example of the way many of these extracellular factors work in normal and tumor cells, we will focus on platelet-derived growth factor (PDGF). A dimer composed of two relatively short protein chains, PDGF has many physiological signaling functions; they include stimulating growth of the endothelial cells that line blood vessels and of connective tissue that contains fibroblasts (the cell type often propagated in tissue culture). As its name implies, PDGF is synthesized and stored in blood platelets, which release it in copious amounts as they form clots; it aids wound healing by prompting the growth of connective tissue cells. This release also creates the abundance of PDGF found in serum. (PDGF and other GFs confer growth-stimulatory properties on serum that make it an essential ingredient in the medium used to propagate cells in culture.)

As we discussed in Chapter 4, the gene that encodes one of the two protein subunits (the B chain) of PDGF is a cellular proto-oncogene, c-sis—the progenitor of the v-sis oncogene of simian sarcoma virus. In the normal platelet–fibroblast relationship, PDGF is produced and released during a specific physiologic event—wounding and blood clot formation—and works by the paracrine mode of action. When simian sarcoma virus infects a fibroblast, however, the viral sis oncogene creates and sustains PDGF production at a high and unrelenting level by the fibroblast itself. The cell releases and then responds to its own PDGF; this autocrine stimulation, which results in cell transformation, no longer depends upon PDGF synthesis by nearby platelets. This situation is repeated in the initially infected fibroblast's descendants, which inherit the chromosomally integrated provirus carrying the v-sis oncogene. Growth of the infected cell is now autoregulated: the fibroblast is making its own GF rather than depending upon neighbors (such as platelets) for growth-promoting instructions. Growth factor autonomy ensues, and excessive growth, promoted by the autocrine route, can result in a tumor cell. The usual interdependency of multiple interacting cell types is disrupted.

Other important elements in this signaling process are the receptor molecules that a cell displays on its surface and uses to detect the presence of PDGF in the environment outside the cell. These receptors bind specifically to extracellular PDGF molecules and ignore the presence of all other GFs that may be in the extracellular space.

A cell that is infected with simian sarcoma virus but lacks cell surface PDGF receptors will not be transformed by the v-sis oncogene. The reason for this is simple: while such a cell may be stimulated by v-sis to secrete large amounts of PDGF, none can bind to the cell surface via PDGF receptors and thereby stimulate growth. This cell will, in effect, be oblivious to the presence of the secreted PDGF. This explains why simian sarcoma virus transforms connective tissue cells like fibroblasts but leaves epithelial cells, which have no PDGF receptors, unaffected.

Several other proto-oncogenes encode secreted proteins that normally influence growth and differentiation through cell surface receptors. Almost always, oncogenic mutations of such genes exaggerate production of the growth factors without altering their molecular structure. The v-sis oncogene does encode a protein whose sequence differs somewhat from the B chain of normal cellular PDGF produced by the c-sis proto-oncogene, but there is no obvious physiological difference between the two proteins. Far more important is the high, unregulated level of PDGF production driven by the viral transcriptional promoter.

A variety of secreted factors may be overproduced by tumor cells deriving from a tissue lineage that usually makes the same factor in well-regulated quantities. T-cell lymphomas, for example, may produce high levels of IL2, the same factor that their normal lymphocyte predecessors release in carefully parceled amounts to autostimulate proliferation as part of the normal immune response. Sometimes growth factor expression by tumor cells is entirely ectopic (out of place), occurring in cell types where it is not usually seen. For example, when a provirus is integrated next to the Wnt-1 proto-oncogene in the chromosomes of mouse mammary tumor virus-infected cells of the breast epithelium, these cells synthesize and secrete a growth factor protein they do not normally produce. Yet they are able to respond to the GF (as demonstrated by excessive growth of the gland), indicating that suitable receptors are on hand; these may be receptors designed to detect proteins made by other members of the Wnt gene family that *are* expressed in the normal mammary gland.

Excessive production of GFs by tumor cells is often the result of mutations in other types of genes, rather than the growth factor genes themselves. In particular, the transforming growth factors (TGF-α and TGF-β) and PDGF are commonly produced by cancer cells without evidence that mutations in the respective growth factor genes are responsible—a situation that presumably reflects distorted regulation of these genes as a secondary result of mutation of other genes that normally regulate growth factor expression indirectly. For example, ras and src oncogenes are known to be able, by unknown means, to turn on high-level expression of the TGF-α and TGF-β genes.

Any overproduced growth factor may influence the growth of the cell that produces it, and it may also stimulate the growth of nearby normal cells. In theory, such a paracrine mechanism may force the growth of normal cells, recruiting them into the proliferating mass of a tumor. In fact, however, the vast majority of cells in actual tumors are members of cell clones that share genetic defects and descend from common ancestor cells; the contribution of paracrine-recruited neighbor cells to such masses appears to be slight.

THE PDGF RECEPTOR AND ITS COUSINS

Aberrations in receptor function represent the next stage at which growth control can be derailed. Inappropriate activation of a receptor molecule may persuade a cell that the receptor's proper ligand (a growth factor, for instance) is in the extracellular space, when in fact none is present. The result may be cell growth in the absence of extracellular stimulation, with consequent growth factor autonomy. To understand this, we turn to the PDGF receptor molecule.

PDGF receptors are large protein chains, over 800 amino acids long. Inserted into the outer (plasma) membrane of many types of cells, about half of the chain is exposed to the outside environment and the other half is bathed in the cytoplasm. The receptor is anchored in this position by a small segment of the protein called the transmembrane domain, composed of water-aversive (hydrophobic) amino acid residues that favor the fatty environment of the membrane. The cytoplasmic portion of the receptor is a protein-tyrosine kinase, recognizable from the resemblance of

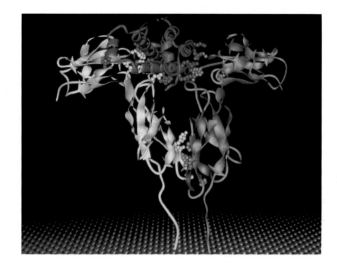

The interaction of human growth hormone with the extracellular portion of its receptor, analyzed by X-ray crystallography. Two receptor molecules (shown in different colors) are driven into a dimeric state by binding to the growth hormone protein.

its sequence to src and src-related proteins and documented by direct tests of its enzymatic activity, which demonstrate its ability to attach phosphate groups to the tyrosine residues of other proteins and even to some of its own residues.

Each cell that expresses PDGF receptors has about 10,000 such molecules, although occasionally the number can approach one million per cell. These receptors are interspersed among many other transmembrane proteins that also protrude from the cell surface and are designed to sense soluble factors other than PDGF or to make contact with the extracellular matrix.

The crucial first step in receptor action—perception of the factor—involves a direct

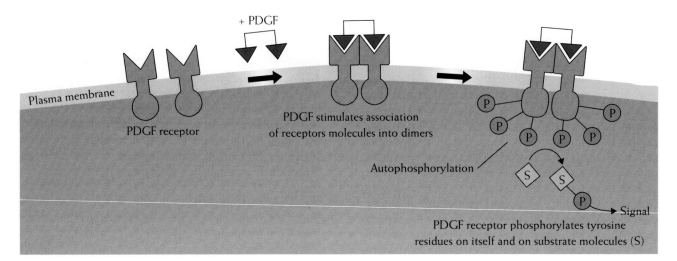

+ PDGF

Plasma membrane

PDGF receptor

PDGF stimulates association
of receptors molecules into dimers

Autophosphorylation

Signal

PDGF receptor phosphorylates tyrosine
residues on itself and on substrate molecules (S)

Activation of the PDGF receptor by the mitogen, PDGF.

physical association between PDGF (the ligand) and the receptor, which in turn depends
upon an adequate concentration of the ligand
in the extracellular fluid. The association is
highly specific: the receptor does not sense
other polypeptide growth factors, even when
present at much higher concentrations than
PDGF, and PDGF will not bind to receptors
for those other factors. This binding specificity, dictated by the amino acid sequences of
the factor and receptor, is embodied in the
three-dimensional folded structures of these
two molecules. Although the precise shapes of
PDGF and its receptor have not yet been determined by X-ray crystallography, the known
structures of analogous proteins allow us to
predict the conformations of these two interac-
tive molecules. It is anticipated that one surface of the folded PDGF molecule fits into a
contoured web of the external arm of its receptor, like a hand into a glove.

Binding of the PDGF ligand by its receptor
is meaningless to the cell unless the event is

communicated to the cell's interior. Three
changes seem to occur within seconds after the
PDGF receptor binds to PDGF: (1) dimerization; (2) activation of intracellular enzymatic
activity; and (3) phosphorylation of tyrosine
residues in the receptor and in other sub-
strates. First, individual receptor molecules,
originally scattered throughout the plasma
membrane as single units, associate as pairs
(homodimers), presumably as a result of affin-
ity with the dimeric PDGF molecules, which
may bridge two receptor molecules, drawing
them together. Next, the dimerization of the
extracellular domains of two receptors brings
their connected cytoplasmic domains into close
contact. Each receptor carries a hitherto silent
tyrosine kinase that now phosphorylates tyrosine residues on the other's chain. These
phosophorylations appear to activate the full
catalytic powers of the kinases; in effect, the
two kinases turn each other on. Finally, the
kinases are now poised to phosphorylate yet
other proteins in the cytoplasm and, in doing

so, transmit growth-promoting information to them. As we will discuss shortly, the PDGF receptor may be able to release several distinctive chemical signals into the cytoplasm by altering several different kinds of substrate molecules.

This scheme represents a powerful means for passing signals through the plasma membrane, and a number of other growth factor receptors are built on a virtually identical plan. In each case, a large extracellular portion of the receptor can recognize and bind a designated factor with great sensitivity and specificity, and in response a protein-tyrosine kinase domain on the cytoplasmic side of the plasma membrane becomes catalytically active. It is striking to find that so many receptors communicate through tyrosine phosphorylation, when only about 0.1 percent of the phospho-amino acid in total cellular protein is phospho-tyrosine.

Among the receptors known to behave in this way are those for insulin (which has growth-promoting actions in addition to its better known roles in sugar uptake and metabolism); for factors that govern the differentiation and growth of blood cells (for example, a blood stem cell factor); for several closely related fibroblast growth factors (FGFs); for the nerve growth factor (NGF) and other less well characterized nerve cell stimulants; and for the epidermal growth factor (EGF) and TGF-α, two proteins that use the same receptor. There are also several other proteins designed like the PDGF receptor for which specific ligands, and hence physiological functions, are not yet known.

These complex molecules create a vulnerability. If they are damaged or overexpressed in certain ways, their tyrosine kinase domains may become activated even in the absence of extracellular ligand. This inappropriate firing has been observed most often in two cousins of the PDGF receptor: the EGF receptor and its close relative, the neu (erb B-2) receptor. This vulnerability first became clear when the structure of the erbB oncogene, carried by avian erythroblastosis virus, turned out to be a truncated version of the normal chicken EGF receptor gene. We now know that the EGF receptor can be converted into a potent oncoprotein by lopping off most of its extracellular domain. The tyrosine kinase domain of the remnant molecule then fires continuously, forcing cell growth in total independence of the presence or absence of EGF. For this reason, the normal EGF receptor gene is considered a proto-oncogene, sometimes termed c-erbB.

There are still more ways to turn on receptor kinases without the requisite ligand. The erb B-2 (neu) protein becomes converted into a powerful transforming protein in rats when a

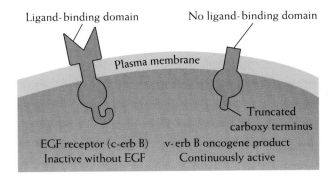

Normal (unstimulated) and mutant forms of the EGF receptor; the latter is encoded by the oncogene of avian erythroblastosis virus, derived from the normal EGF receptor gene.

Varieties of Transmembrane Receptors

Receptors built on the PDGF model are most often implicated in cancer, but there are also many other kinds of cell surface receptors, including several with important roles in normal and abnormal growth. It is in their cytoplasmic, signal-emitting regions that their functional diversity becomes most apparent. The receptor for the extracellular factor that usually restrains growth (TFG-β) has a protein kinase activity that adds phosphate to serine or threonine residues on target proteins, rather than to tyrosine residues (as on the mitogen receptors). Other presumptive receptors (for which ligands are not yet identified) remove bound phosphate from tyrosines of the target proteins rather than adding it, thereby reversing the effects of the mitogen receptors. Yet others convert the nucleotide GTP to a compound known as cyclic GMP. A very large group of receptors, including those for many of the cytokines that govern the growth and differentiation of hematopoietic cells, have relatively short cytoplasmic tails without apparent enzymatic capacity. How might a signal issue from such receptors? In a few cases, the cytoplasmic portion is known to make contact with the src-related tyrosine kinases, stimulating their activity; other cytoplasmic proteins that might form such bipartite complexes with receptors are now being sought.

An unrelated but common group of cell surface receptors are constructed from protein chains that pass through the plasma membrane not just once, but seven times. These so-called serpentine receptors respond to many kinds of signals that are beyond our discussion here: odors, light, and a huge variety of hormones. A few of the serpentine receptors have been reported to contribute to cancerous growth when produced at unusually high concentrations. Most of the serpentine receptors communicate with the interior of a cell through contacts with tripartite G proteins, composed of three subunits; of these, the alpha subunit is (like ras proteins) active when bound to GTP and silenced when GTP is converted to GDP; the amino acid sequences of those subunits are closely related to the sequences of ras products. In several kinds of human cancers (especially carcinomas of the pituitary and adrenal glands), mutant alpha subunits occur with physiological properties analogous to those encountered with mutant ras proteins; they, too, are stuck in the "on" position. This is especially interesting because the downstream target of these tripartite G proteins is known (unlike the target for ras proteins); it is the enzyme adenylate cyclase, which converts ATP to the second messenger cyclic AMP (see page 136), a potent growth stimulator in these specialized cell types.

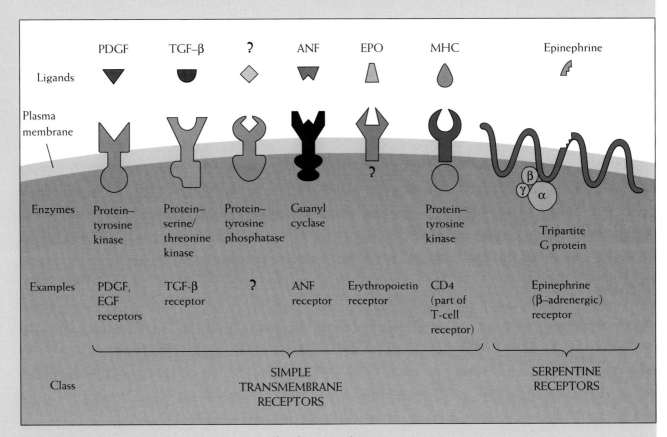

Varieties of receptors for signal transmission across the plasma membrane.

single amino acid residue in its transmembrane domain is replaced because of a point mutation in its encoding gene. The resulting mutant receptors form stable dimers, and their associated tyrosine kinases are placed in a permanently activated state.

In human tumor cells, this same receptor protein may be prompted to signal simply by being overexpressed—tenfold or more above usual amounts. The excess receptor molecules seem to dimerize spontaneously; they may also make a cell hypersensitive to amounts of ligand that, on their own, would be too low to induce a growth response. Excessive erb B-2 (neu) receptor protein—seen in many human breast, stomach, and ovarian carcinomas—may play an important role in promoting aggressive metastatic growth.

All these alterations in the amounts and structures of receptors have the same result: they enable tyrosine kinase receptors to fire in the absence of amounts of growth factor ligand normally required to trigger growth. In each case, the outcome is that the proliferation of the cell no longer depends upon signaling from extracellular sources.

MODES OF CYTOPLASMIC SIGNALING

By far the most complex stage in the signaling process involves the array of cytoplasmic proteins that normally receive messages from ligand-activated receptors and pass them along a variety of pathways. Each of these proteins is said to be a transducer of signals in the sense that it receives an incoming (afferent) signal from a growth factor receptor, processes it, and releases an outgoing (efferent) signal to the next protein down the line. These signal transducers may also act as amplifiers, receiving a small incoming signal and, in response, releasing a much larger flow of outgoing signals. Cell transformation may ensue when signal transducers suffer structural changes that cause them to emit downstream signals even without prompting by their usual upstream controllers—the ligand-activated receptors.

Once again, the processes triggered by PDGF prove enlightening. A large number of cytoplasmic proteins acquire phosphate groups on tyrosines within seconds after PDGF is added to the extracellular environment. Many, perhaps all, of these proteins may be phosphorylated directly by the PDGF receptor kinase domain; several become physically attached to the receptor protein, and their identities provide clues to the downstream signaling cascades that the receptor triggers. We will briefly indicate the nature of this complex cytoplasmic circuitry by examining four of the proteins that associate directly with the cytoplasmic domain of the PDGF receptor following ligand binding: phospholipase C (PLC); phosphatidyl inositol kinase (PI3 kinase); pp60^{src} (the protein encoded by the src proto-oncogene); and ras GTPase activating protein (ras-GAP). Each provides a clue about the radiating pathways that the receptor uses to activate cell growth.

Our most detailed account follows PLC and PI3 kinase, enzymes that help create potent intracellular hormones termed second messengers. These messengers are low-molecular-weight compounds synthesized near the inner

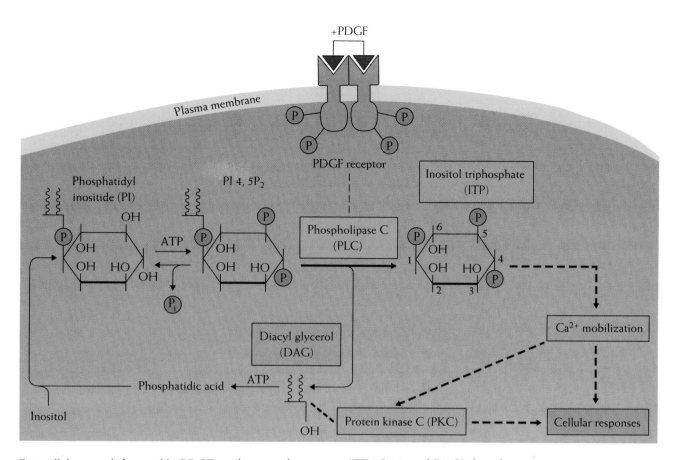

Extracellular growth factors, like PDGF, produce second messengers (ITP, Ca²⁺, and DAG) through the effects of phospholipase C upon phosphatidyl inositol turnover. The second messengers, in turn, affect enzymes such as protein kinase C.

surface of the cell membrane for dispatch to distant sites in the cell, where they elicit specific responses. In this way, localized receptor changes can produce global alterations in the cell. Important second messengers include cyclic nucleotides like cyclic AMP (adenosine monophosphate) and cyclic GMP (guanosine monophosphate), inositol triphosphate (ITP), diacyl glycerol (DAG), and even calcium ions (Ca^{2+}). Each of these molecules is normally kept at very low cytoplasmic concentrations that may be raised briefly but transiently by one or another ligand-activated receptor.

We concentrate here on the inositol pathway, which is tightly associated with growth stimulation. As seen in the flowchart, at the top of this path are phosphatidyl inositides (PIs), which are stored by the cell among the lipids that form the plasma membrane. By modifying and then breaking down these

The SH2 Paradigm

Transmission of signals for growth control often depends upon the ability of one protein to structurally modify a second; in effect, to communicate with it. Such communication can occur through subtle and readily reversible enzymatic reactions—for example, the addition or removal of a phosphate residue, or the conversion of protein-bound GTP to GDP, which can later be replaced once again by GTP. But often signaling is not enzymatic, instead consisting of transient contact between two proteins. Such contacts as the binding of a growth factor to its membrane-associated receptor seem relatively simple, regulated mainly by availability of the two reactants. Others, like those involving transcription factors (page 141), require multiple interactions: the factors pair, then bind to certain DNA sequences, and only then contact RNA polymerase to stimulate transcription.

A short sequence of 100 amino acids—the SH2 domain—is used to bind partner proteins by many proteins implicated in signaling growth. The SH2 (src homology-2) domain on one protein will recognize and bind to a phosphorylated tyrosine (and the surrounding amino acids) of its partner; it will ignore the partner if the critical tyrosine is not phosphorylated. When the PDGF receptor is activated by binding its ligand (PDGF), the receptor autophosphorylates, creating a number of phosphotyrosine groups. Each of these now acts as a magnet to attract and bind a partner protein containing an SH2 domain. Among these partners are the src protein, for which the SH2 sequence was named; other partners are phospholipase C, PI3 kinase, and ras GTPase activating protein (ras-GAP). Once bound to the receptor via its SH2 domain, each of these proteins can release further cytoplasmic signals, either because it also can now be phosphorylated by the receptor's kinase or because it undergoes some subtle change in protein folding.

---

membrane building blocks, the cell can create smaller molecules that are potent second messengers.

The PDGF receptor binds, phosphorylates, and activates one of the PI kinases that adds phosphates to the inositol ring. The biochemical fate of the product of this PI kinase is not yet known, but genetic experiments indicate that it must have a central role in driving a cell into the growth cycle.

Phosphorylated PIs may be converted into the active second messenger molecules ITP and DAG when they are cleaved by the PLC enzyme—one of the proteins that associates with the PDGF receptor and is phosphorylated and stimulated by it. ITP, diffusing through the

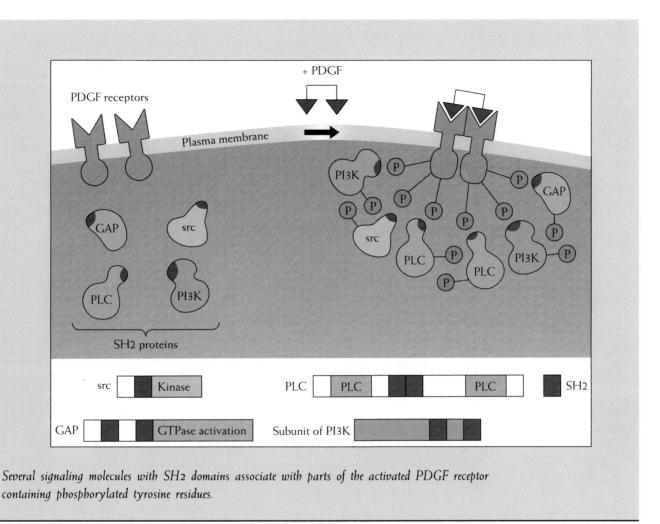

Several signaling molecules with SH2 domains associate with parts of the activated PDGF receptor containing phosphorylated tyrosine residues.

cytoplasm, provokes the release of Ca^{2+} ions from membranous sacks where they are usually sequestered; the rapid rise in intracellular calcium in turn activates several dozen responding enzymes.

The other PI cleavage product—DAG—collaborates with the released Ca^{2+} to activate yet another centrally important growth-regulat-ing enzyme, protein kinase C (PKC), which phosphorylates threonine and serine residues on dozens of target proteins, presumably modifying their activity. We now see how a small number of enzymes acting in concert with the receptor can elicit a multitude of responses at distant sites in the cell. This same PKC enzyme is a receptor for the tumor-promoting

The Quintessential Second Messenger

yclic AMP (cAMP) was the first molecule to be carefully studied as a second messenger in signaling pathways, mainly those stimulated by hormones that affect cell metabolism. Although only sporadically associated with growth control and cancer, cyclic AMP exemplifies how a small, diffusible molecule can transfer information received at the plasma membrane to alter programs of gene expression in the nucleus. In contrast, the biochemical signaling mechanisms of the small molecules that serve as second messengers to control growth (for example, diacyl glycerol and Ca^{2+}) have not been as crisply defined.

Cyclic AMP is the pivotal link between signals from many serpentine cell surface receptors (page 131) and certain transcription factors (page 141). This signaling pathway is controlled by the concentration of cyclic AMP, as determined by the behavior of two counterbalancing enzymes: one that converts ATP into cyclic AMP in a single step, and one that converts cyclic AMP back to the noncyclic form of AMP (a substrate for the generation of more ATP). In the presence of their extracellular ligands (such as the hormone epinephrine), most serpentine receptors stimulate the former pathway. The resulting rapid increase in

Hormones stimulate the production of cAMP via serpentine receptors, tripartite G proteins (page 130), and adenylate cyclase.

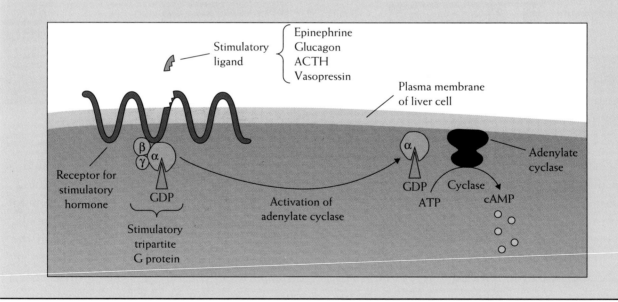

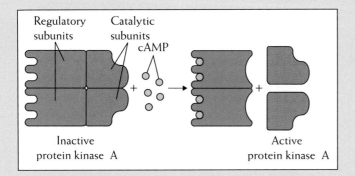

Regulatory subunits   Catalytic subunits   cAMP

Inactive protein kinase A   Active protein kinase A

Cyclic AMP stimulates protein kinase A by removing inhibitory (regulatory) subunits.

partite G proteins or overexpressed serpentine receptors may yield abnormally high levels of cyclic AMP, leading to growth deregulation. These changes can be useful in diagnosis and could provide future targets for therapeutic intervention.

cyclic AMP concentration has a dramatic effect: the second messenger, which is freely diffusible throughout the cell, activates an abundant kinase—the cyclic AMP-dependent protein kinase (PK-A)—that in turn phosphorylates serines and threonines in various target proteins. This activation occurs in an interesting way: cyclic AMP binds to an inhibitory protein normally complexed to PK-A, causing it to liberate active enzyme. Among the important targets for PK-A are transcription factors whose ability to bind to DNA and alter the readout of certain genes depends upon phosphorylation. A large collection of cellular genes is known to be regulated by these cyclic AMP-dependent transcription factors.

Cyclic AMP deregulation does not appear to be a major factor in most neoplasms. But in certain tumors, mutant tri-

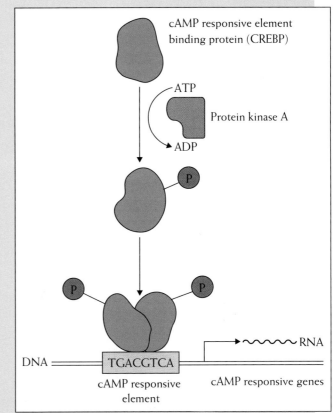

cAMP responsive element binding protein (CREBP)

ATP

Protein kinase A

ADP

P

P   P

DNA   TGACGTCA   RNA

cAMP responsive element   cAMP responsive genes

Activated protein kinase A phosphorylates a subclass of transcription factors; this is the mechanism by which cyclic AMP regulates gene expression.

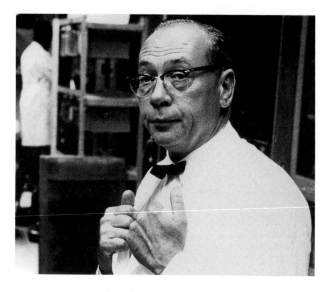

Earl Sutherland, the discoverer of cyclic AMP.

phorbol esters, which mimic DAG action and play a key role in skin carcinogenesis, as the following chapter will show.

The association of the normal src protein with the PDGF receptor suggests that src's enzymatic activity may be regulated by the receptor kinase. Normal src protein is tightly controlled: its activity as a tyrosine kinase is latent until activated by incoming signals, such as those provided by PDGF. The contrasting v-src protein, made by the Rous sarcoma virus, is structurally altered so that it is constantly active. The potential importance of c-src protein is indicated by the profound changes in cell behavior that its aberrant v-src cousin induces in RSV-transformed cells. The precise

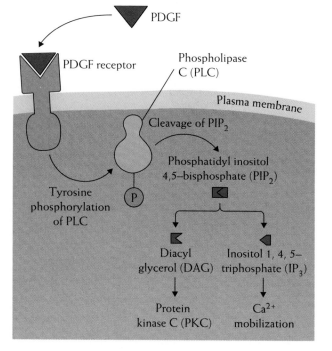

The activated PDGF receptor contacts, phosphorylates, and thereby activates PLC.

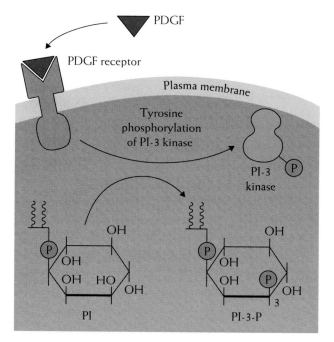

The activated PDGF receptor contacts, phosphorylates, and thereby activates PI3 kinase.

role of the c-src protein in conveying signals from the PDGF receptor has yet to be clearly defined.

Another critical branch of the receptor's downstream signaling pathway is revealed by the presence of the ras-GAP protein in complexes with the PDGF receptor. Ras-GAP is a multifunctional protein that converses with the receptor through one of its domains and with the ras signaling pathway through another. Plugging into the ras pathway, the receptor gains access to one of the most potent regulatory circuits in the cell.

Aberrant forms of the ras protein, which we described in some biochemical detail in Chapter 4, are found in 25 to 30 percent of human tumors. Like a number of other signaling molecules in the cell, the ras protein (termed here p21^{ras}) exists in two states, active and inactive. The transition between these two forms is not demarcated by chemical modification of p21^{ras}, however, such as the attach-

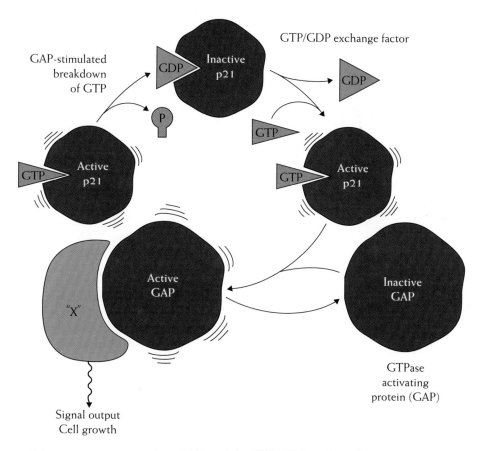

The effects of the ras GTPase activating protein (ras-GAP) and the GTP–GDP exchange factor upon signaling by p21^{ras}.

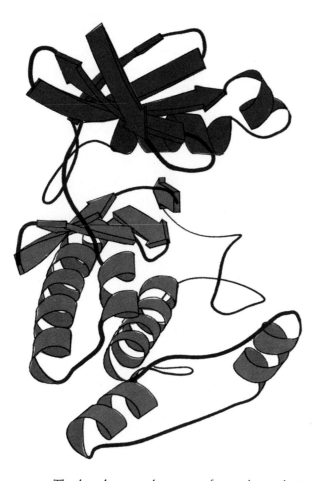

The three-dimensional structure of a catalytic subunit of protein kinase A (PKA). ATP is bound and the transfer of phosphate to target proteins takes place in the cleft between the upper and lower portions of the molecule.

ment and removal of chemically bound phosphate groups. Instead, the signaling state of p21^{ras} is indicated by the alternative binding of the nucleotides GDP and GTP.

P21^{ras} binds GDP when it is inactive. In a fashion that is still poorly understood, ligand-activated growth factor receptors force p21^{ras} to release its captive GDP molecule. A GTP molecule replaces it, switching p21^{ras} to an active, signal-emitting mode. Within seconds, however, p21^{ras} breaks down its bound GTP into GDP, causing p21^{ras} to return to its inactive mode and thereby ensuring that only a carefully rationed pulse of excitatory signal is passed from p21^{ras} to its downstream partners, which in turn activate parts of the cell's growth program. Presumably, the association of ras-GAP with the activated PDGF receptor has some influence on this process, since ras-GAP is able to turn off ras signaling by promoting the breakdown of GTP to GDP.

The mutant oncogenic p21^{ras} molecules found in many cancers have suffered subtle structural alterations: replacement of single residues in the 12th or 61st position of their amino acid chains. The mutant oncogenic form functions like the normal p21^{ras} molecule, but it is defective in one important respect. No longer able to convert its bound GTP to GDP, even when brought in contact with ras-GAP, it lacks the ability to shut itself off. As a direct consequence, it is trapped for extended periods in its excited state and floods the cytoplasm with an unrelenting stream of growth-stimulating signals.

We have seen, using the example of these four proteins, how the interior of a cancer cell may receive potent growth-stimulatory signals, even without encountering any mitogenic GF. The resulting autonomy derives from the fact that the growth program of the cancer cell is dictated by mutant components of its internal machinery, not by signals arriving from outside the cell. (Still missing in this scenario are precise descriptions of how GF receptors regulate p21^{ras} activity and how activated p21^{ras} induces the cell to grow.) These diverse biomechanical mechanisms—kinase activation, protein–protein association, altered lipid metabolism, and second messenger production—constitute many of the cytoplasmic consequences of the activation of growth factor receptors. But many of the ultimate targets of growth-controlling molecules reside in the nucleus: the machinery for gene expression, DNA synthesis, and separation of duplicated chromosomes into daughter nuclei. How do cytoplasmic signaling pathways finally reach the molecules that replicate the genome and make RNA transcripts of cellular genes? How do these nuclear processes become deregulated by oncogenic proteins?

TRANSCRIPTION FACTORS

A number of important controllers of nuclear processes might, in principle, serve as targets for oncogenic deregulation. In practice, however, the proteins that affect transcriptional activity are most often implicated in the cancer process. Many proteins appear to influence directly how often specific genes (or sets of genes) are transcribed: without the intervention of these so-called transcription factors, their responder genes will not be read out into RNA copies and hence will remain unexpressed and biologically silent. At least three kinds of interactions, working in concert, are central to the ability of transcription factors to turn on or off the expression of specific responder genes:

(1) DNA binding; (2) dimerization of transcription factors; and (3) interaction with the transcription complex.

Each transcription factor must be able to target the particular set of genes that it regulates. To do so, it must recognize and bind to a short DNA sequence, generally about eight to ten base pairs long, that identifies a gene as being subject to control by the factor. The binding reaction may require direct contact between the factor and DNA, or the factor may be part of a multiprotein complex, some other component of which contacts the DNA sequence directly. The recognition sequences are usually within a few hundred base pairs from the given gene's start site for transcription, but they may be thousands or even tens of thousands of base pairs away and still affect the transcription rate. Furthermore, each gene may have recognition sequences for several distinct factors that collaborate to turn it on or off.

Many transcription factors are found in two-protein complexes; the partners may be identical (homodimers) or different (heterodimers). Amino acid motifs known as leucine zippers and helix-loop-helix regions allow elaborate intertwining of the two pairing protein chains. Some transcription factors are able to form dimers with several kinds of partners, yielding different complexes with differing affinities for binding sites in DNA—a variation that may allow a diverse collection of genes to be regulated in both directions by these dimerizing factors.

To alter the rate of transcription, the factors must also make contact with the enzyme complex featuring RNA polymerase that initi-

Regulation of Transcription Factors

T he control of gene transcription, one of the greatest problems in modern biology, is central to an understanding of cancer. Consider, first of all, the magnitude of the problem. The rates of RNA synthesis must be regulated for each of around 100,000 different genes in every cell type. It must be possible to vary the rates in response to calls for growth or differentiation. The complex pattern of regulation must also take into account the fact that the vast majority of genes are read by the same enzyme, RNA polymerase II.

The vigor with which any gene is copied by this polymerase is governed by at least two components: the varied collection of short DNA sequences (recognition signals for transcription factors) near the beginning of each gene, and the availability of active factors. Hundreds of genes encode transcription factors, and the effective number is made even larger by combination: most of these proteins can form heter-

odimers with several proteins, and each pair may have different specificities.

Several devices vary the abundance of active factors. Proteins that compose some factors may be constantly present yet require some chemical modification (for example, the addition of phosphate groups)

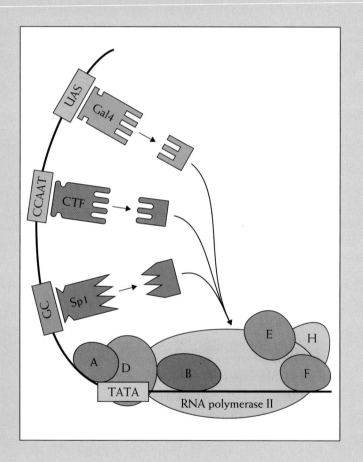

Transcription factors (GAL4, CTF, Sp1) bind to specific DNA sequences (called UAS, CCAT, CG) and interact through adapter proteins with the enzymatic machinery (RNA polymerase II and associated proteins A–H) positioned at the start site for transcription (near TATA).

or the displacement of a bound inhibitor to become active. Others are, in effect, receptors for fat-soluble hormones, such as steroid or thyroid hormones, which can enter a cell by slipping through the plasma membrane. When such transcription factors-cum-receptors bind to their ligands, the factors are refolded, allowing them to bind DNA and influence transcription rates. The activities of yet other transcription factors are determined simply by their concentrations in cells: the influence of such factors rises and falls dramatically, controlled by the expression of the genes encoding them.

From a gene's DNA sequence, it is often possible to recognize and predict at least several of the transcription factors that are likely to influence its transcription into RNA. Conversely, a transcription factor's amino acid sequence will often suggest the kinds of proteins with which it will form dimers, the DNA sequences to which it will bind, the domain that it uses to stimulate RNA polymerase, and whether its activity will be regulated by hormones, inhibitors, or phosphorylation.

Especially vivid among these motifs are the amino acid sequences that bring proteins together as heterodimers. One such motif, an array of amino acids punctuated every seven residues with a greasy, protrud-

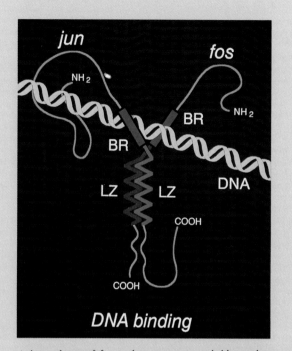

DNA binding

A heterodimer of fos and jun proteins is held together by a leucine zipper region (LZ), binds to its recognition site in DNA by its basic region (BR), and then enhances or represses transcription by RNA polymerase.

ing leucine side chain, is called a leucine zipper. Two proteins with such domains can wrap around each other; the adjacent chains then form two arms capable of embracing DNA with an appropriate sequence, while another portion of the factor makes additional contacts that affect the RNA polymerase transcription rate.

ates RNA chains at the start site for transcription. Clues to the nature of this interaction are available from studies of bacterial transcription factors, which touch a portion of the RNA polymerase molecule; direct contacts of this type are also likely to occur in animal cells. This is possible even when the recognition sequences for the factors are located far from the start site, because factors bound to distant regulatory sites can be brought close to the start site by bending the DNA into a loop.

How are the activities of transcription factors within the nucleus regulated by extracellular signals, and how is this regulation upset in cancer cells? The most dramatic cases are provided by three classes of factors, products of the myc, fos, and jun gene families. In serum-deprived, resting cells, these genes are silent and their proteins—each a transcription factor—are virtually undetectable in the cell. When PDGF is added, levels of fos and jun factors skyrocket within minutes and myc follows suit in an hour or two.

Once they accumulate in sufficient amounts in the nucleus, each of these factors can activate expression of a large bank of responder genes. In fact, a jun and a fos protein molecule join to form a heterodimeric transcription factor that binds to a sequence present in the control regions of many genes. Myc associates with its own partner, named max, whose concentrations within the cell are held constant; the myc:max pair then binds to genes displaying a specific DNA sequence, presumably activating their transcription. It is thought that the genes responding to fos, jun, and myc factors yield many of the protein products that in aggregate are required to form an actively grow-ing cell. In this sense, these three transcription factors can be viewed as master regulators of cell growth.

Precisely how growth factor receptors acting at the cell periphery communicate with and turn on myc, fos, and jun expression remains a mystery. One thing, however, is already very clear: in many cancer cells, the induction of these genes and the transcription factors that they encode no longer depends upon growth factor stimulation. Now these genes may be expressed steadily, independent of normal growth factor control.

The capacity of genes like myc, fos, and jun that encode transcription factors to promote neoplastic growth has been amply documented (Chapter 4). In human cells of Burkitt's lymphoma, for instance, the control sequences normally regulating myc expression have been removed by chromosomal translocation and replaced by control sequences from an antibody gene on another chromosome. The antibody control sequences sustain myc expression that is totally independent of normal extracellular regulating signals. This steadily expressed myc gene has become a myc oncogene. In the genome of avian myelocytomatosis virus, where myc was first discovered, its expression is driven by a strong retroviral transcription regulator. Similarly, in certain avian lymphomas, retrovirus integration into the chromosomal myc proto-oncogene usurps normal myc regulation by placing myc expression under control of the provirus.

Regardless of mechanism, myc expression remains constantly elevated and, accordingly, can orchestrate active cell growth even when the cell is deprived of outside GFs. The fos and jun genes follow this basic pattern. Each can become a potent oncogene when its expression is placed under the control of a foreign regulator—a steady, GF-independent controller like a retroviral transcription promoter. Once again the uncoupling of intracellular signaling from extracellular stimuli results in growth factor autonomy.

Escape from Growth Inhibition

Growth factor independence is not the only way that evolving cancer cells can be deregulated—they can also lose responsiveness to the external signals that normally serve to *inhibit* cell growth. These negative signals appear to be equally important in choreographing the finely balanced growth of normal cells. As Chapter 5 argued, a cell that has lost a tumor suppressor gene and its protein product has lost its brakes—a situation potentially as dangerous as the stuck accelerator created by an activated oncogene.

While much is known about the biochemical mechanisms of action of oncoproteins, rather little is understood about how growth-inhibitory proteins act biochemically. Perhaps the simplest mechanism involves interrupting the cell's progression through its growth cycle. The product of the retinoblastoma gene is thought to block emergence of the cell from the G1 phase, in part by binding to—and thereby inactivating—a transcription factor

that governs the reading out of several genes whose products are necessary for further growth. A related mechanism appears to explain the growth-retarding effects of another tumor suppressor gene, the Wilms' tumor gene (WT-1). The product of this gene is a transcription factor that binds to the same DNA sequence recognized by another factor, called Egr-1. But while Egr-1 promotes growth by augmenting transcription, the competing WT-1 may interfere with growth by repressing transcription of the same gene. Thus deficiencies of either of these two tumor suppressor genes—Rb or WT-1—can lead, by different mechanisms, to the excessive activity of transcription factors that promote growth when not restrained by Rb or WT-1 proteins.

Addition of the growth-inhibitory factor TGF-β to culture media similarly induces many cell types to cease growth in the G1 phase. Like the mitogenic factors, TGF-β binds to a cell surface transmembrane receptor. Unlike the growth-promoting receptors (such as that of PDGF), the TGF-β receptor contains in its cytoplasmic domain a serine-threonine kinase that appears to emit growth-inhibitory signals into the cell cytoplasm. The growth of normal retinal cells is very sensitive to inhibition by TGF-β, but retinoblastoma cells grow well in its presence. These tumor cells seem to have escaped the suppressive influence of this factor, thereby gaining a growth advantage in a tissue where TGF-β is present, by a simple trick: they shut off TGF-β receptor expression and become oblivious to the factor. (The connection between receptor shutdown and the inactivation of Rb gene expression in these cells is still unclear.)

The Ubiquity of Signaling Pathways

T he steps in growth control described in this chapter have been pieced together largely by studying the biochemical properties of a tiny fraction of the many proteins present in any cell. Hyperactive forms of these proteins, the products of mutant proto-oncogenes, can disrupt normal growth regulation, suggesting that they activate some signaling pathway. But much stronger evidence for the existence of the pathways we have sketched—and for their importance in diverse kinds of signaling—has emerged from an unexpected quarter: the study of genes affecting the development of specialized organs in experimentally malleable organisms, such as the fruit fly (*Drosophila melanogaster*) and a roundworm (*Caenorhabitis elegans*).

Several *Drosophila* mutants fail to produce one of the eight photoreceptor cells in

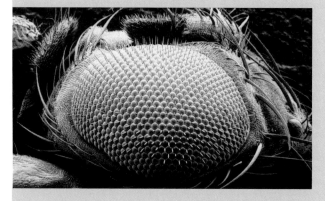

The geometrical array of the elements (ommatidia) in the eye of a normal Drosophila.

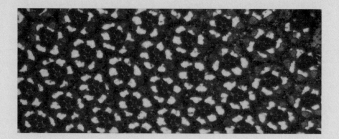

Cross-sections of the ommatidia in the eye of a normal Drosophila *show six retinal photoreceptor cells surrounding the seventh cell* (R7).

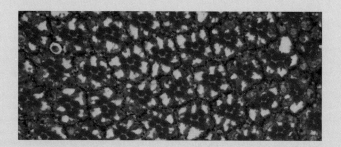

In "sevenless" mutants (and others with the same phenotype), the R7 cell is missing from each ommatidium.

the eye. The absence of this cell (R7) was initially correlated with a defect in a gene called sevenless (sev). The sev product, a transmembrane protein with a cytoplasmic tyrosine kinase activity, resembles a growth factor receptor, like the PDGF receptor. To issue a signal, the sev protein must bind a ligand encoded by another gene (called "bride of sevenless," or boss). Several other proteins form a signaling pathway from the sev receptor on the cell surface to genes ultimately regulated by the boss-initiated signal. Amazingly, these proteins are also part of proposed pathways for growth control in mammalian cells: a ras protein; two proteins that regulate the amount of GTP bound to ras (GAP and a GDP–GTP exchange factor); and a transcription factor.

Equally astounding parallels exist between mammalian growth control and the development of the vulva, site of sperm entry, in the worm *C. elegans*. Several genes have been implicated: multiple vulvae appear when the genes are hyperactive, and no vulva is present when they are deficient. The products of these genes have been identified and placed in sequence. The process is initiated by a single cell that produces an extracellular factor related to EGF and TGF-α; the receptor for this signal on adjacent cells is a single transmembrane protein with a tyrosine kinase domain, resembling the EGF receptor; subsequent components in the pathway are an SH2-containing protein, a ras protein, and a protein kinase specific for serine and threonine residues (closely related to the kinase encoded by the raf proto-oncogene).

Such genetic findings resoundingly confirm the growth regulatory mechanisms being worked out biochemically in cultured mammalian cells and offer new opportuni-

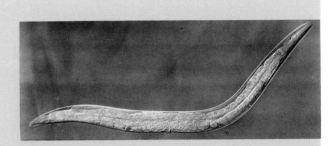

A normal adult nematode (C. elegans); these worms are hermaphrodites, possessing both male and female germ cells. Note the single vulva (ventral surface).

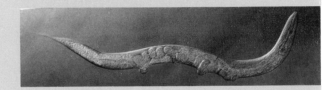

This C. elegans *mutant is unable to form any vulva.*

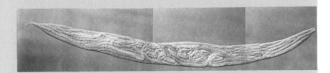

This C. elegans *mutant forms multiple vulvae (ventral surface).*

ties to manipulate the interacting components of the pathways. In addition, they show vividly that these signaling pathways developed early in metazoan evolution—perhaps a billion years ago—and have been adapted for a variety of uses since then.

OTHER WAYS TO RESTRICT GROWTH

At least three other mechanisms ensure that cell proliferation does not exceed the needs of a normal tissue: (1) promotion of cell differentiation by tumor suppressor genes; (2) limitation of the total number of cell generations before senescence; and (3) programmed cell death. Like the cell cycle blocks, these mechanisms may also become subverted during tumor progression, freeing the cancer cell to grow unimpeded.

In an embryo, cells are assigned to particular developmental lineages, which places severe constraints upon their fate. As cells proceed toward full differentiation, they usually lose their ability to divide. For this reason, excessive proliferation can usually be avoided if ap-

propriate numbers of cells are encouraged to proceed toward end-stage differentiation. Most cancer cells resemble relatively immature, undifferentiated cells in the organs in which they have arisen and hence appear to have an unlimited capacity to replicate.

Some tumor suppressor genes may normally limit cell growth by their ability to aid and promote differentiation. The erbA gene product—the nuclear receptor for thyroid hormone—is one example. When the avian erythroblastosis virus enters chicken red-blood-cell precursors, an altered form of erbA, specified by the integrated viral genome, interferes with normal erbA function and therefore with the normal progression of these cells into a mature, nongrowing state. The resulting red-blood-cell precursors, perpetually undifferentiated and competent to proliferate, are now

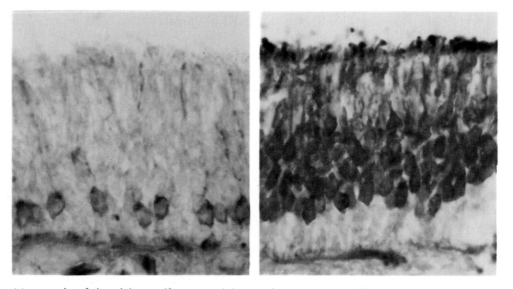

Micrographs of the adult rat olfactory epithelium. Left: Immature, undifferentiated stem cells (stained dark); most cancer cells resemble this type of cell. Right: Mature, differentiated cells in the same tissue (stained dark).

very susceptible to conversion into fully malignant cells.

A second strategy for regulating cell numbers derives from the limited number of divisions of which most cell lineages are normally capable. Rodent fibroblasts, for example, are allotted 30 to 40 doublings and human fibroblasts as many as 60 before they become senescent and stop growing entirely. The p53 gene product appears to play a key role in carrying out this program. It acts in the nucleus, apparently as a transcription factor, to execute some of the steps leading toward this nongrowing state. Mutant, defective forms of p53 block normal p53 function, as we saw in Chapter 5, and therefore the cell's progress to a nongrowing state. The influence of extracellular signals in encouraging cells to senesce is still unresolved.

A final strategy involves the process of programmed cell death, also called apoptosis. A variety of normal developing tissues eliminate improperly developing cells by consigning them to the fate of rapid self-destruction by apoptosis. The p53 gene again seems to play a key role; its mutation prevents the physiologically essential elimination of unneeded cells. Another cancer gene, termed bcl-2, also has a crucial part, at least in the programmed cell death of lymphocytes. The bcl-2 gene is found at the breakpoint in a translocation chromosome in the common human cancer termed follicular B-cell lymphoma. How it interferes with cell death is a mystery: little is known about bcl-2 protein other than its amino acid sequence and its location at a number of cell membranes, including the outer membrane of mitochondria. When transgenic mice express this protein in excessive amounts i[n] lineage, the number of early, und[ifferentiated] cells increases as a consequence [of abnor]mal longevity. Although no tum[ors] result of bcl-2 amplification alone, the e[x]panded cell populations are highly vulnerable to the effects of other oncogenes. Thus, if a myc oncogene is introduced in these animals, B-cell lymphomas occur much more frequently than they would if the bcl-2 transgene were not present.

INTEGRATED CIRCUITS

In this chapter we have described a sometimes bewildering array of molecules present in virtually every part of the cell. Extracellular growth factors such as PDGF provoke growth, whereas others like TGF-β usually restrict it; these opposing effects are mediated through cell surface receptors with distinct biochemical activities. The signals are carried through the cytoplasm by GTP-binding proteins, various protein kinases, enzymes that modify lipids, and second messengers such as Ca^{2+} and cyclic AMP; and the instructions are finally interpreted in the nucleus by transcription factors that set the program for gene expression.

How can we come to grips with the design that governs all these components and activities? Each cell is likely to be continuously bombarded by a combination of extracellular factors, often bearing contradictory messages. Matters do not appear to be any simpler in the cytoplasm, where the diverse signaling mechanisms resemble the parallel circuitry used in computers.

Using New Genetic Methods to Seek the Normal Functions of Proto-Oncogenes

R ecently developed methods for deliberately altering the mouse genome for research purposes are revolutionizing the study of genes and genetic diseases. These techniques depend upon the ability to cultivate stem cells derived from early embryos and manipulate them in culture genetically; these cells retain the capacity to generate

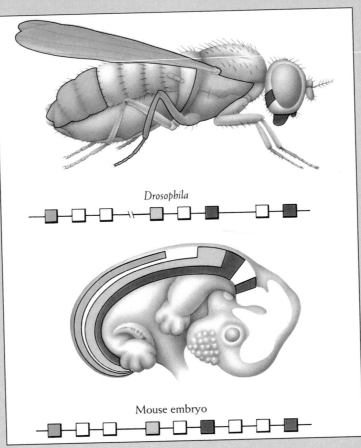

Drosophila

Mouse embryo

Genes encoding certain transcription factors crucial to development are conserved from insects to mammals. As the figure implies, even the chromosomal positions of these genes (squares) and the portions of the animal they influence during development (color coded) may be conserved. These genes, called homeobox genes, are sometimes mutated to form oncogenes, like many other developmentally important genes.

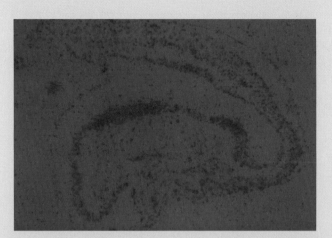

The Wnt-1 proto-oncogene is expressed in the mid-brain region of the developing nervous system of an early mouse embryo. The pink color shows sites at which a labeled probe interacts with Wnt-1 messenger RNA.

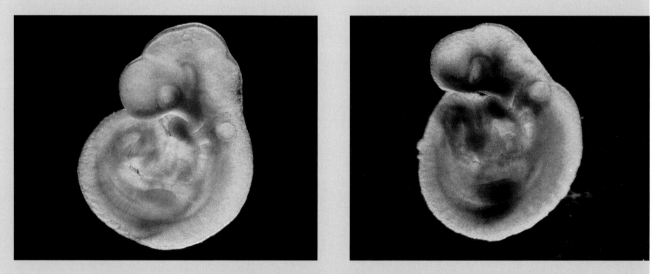

A normal mouse embryo about three-quarters of the way through gestation (left). The large head (spinal cord is at right in both photographs) includes the midbrain and cerebellum, which are missing in an embryo of the same age deprived of the Wnt-1 proto-oncogene (right).

Continued

all cell lineages, including those of the germ cells, when injected into other early embryos. As a consequence, the descendants of these cells (mutated by the researcher's design) will be present in many or all tissues of the developing mouse. If their descendants form the germ cells of the newborn mice, the resulting egg or sperm can transmit the introduced mutation to all subsequent mouse generations.

Genetically altered mice have been used to investigate the consequences of inactivating the genes implicated in cancer. Are individual proto-oncogenes really essential for normal growth and development? Do tumor suppressor genes have functions other than blocking excessive growth? (This question is addressed on page 174.) Does an inherited deficiency of these genes predispose mice to cancer?

Sometimes these experiments provide dramatic evidence for a proto-oncogene's normal function. Consider the example of the Wnt-1 gene, a proto-oncogene that is turned on by a proviral insertion in retrovirus-induced breast cancer in mice. The Wnt-1 gene encodes a secreted protein thought to act like a growth factor for the developing nervous system in the middle phase of embryogenesis. A mouse born without an intact copy of Wnt-1 (inactivated by gene targeting) lacks a complete midbrain and cerebellum—parts of the brain derived from one of the regions in which Wnt-1 is normally expressed. This shows clearly that the Wnt-1 gene, discovered through its involvement in mammary carcinogenesis, is absolutely essential to make major parts of the brain.

Elimination of the src proto-oncogene, expressed in nearly every tissue in mammals, has relatively meager effects. Most tissues remain normal, including those like the brain and blood platelets, where especially high concentrations of src protein are normally found. (The capacity of most cells to tolerate loss of src protein is presumably explained by the presence of very similar proteins encoded by other members of the src gene family.) But one cell type, the osteoclast, a cell responsible for reabsorption of bone tissue during the continuous remodeling of bone, is malfunctional. As a result, affected animals form excessive amounts of bone, a debilitating condition known as osteopetrosis.

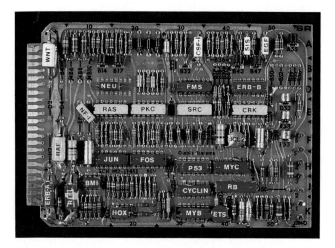

A fanciful model of the circuitry involved in cell signaling, with the extracellular factors on top and the transcription factors at the bottom.

To be sure, some patterns have emerged. A range of genetic and biochemical approaches testify to certain sequences of events in the circuitry: tyrosine kinases usually act upstream of ras proteins, which in turn act upstream of certain serine-threonine kinases. But there is also considerable evidence for divergent, redundant, and parallel processing of information. Individual receptors (like the one for PDGF) interact with numerous signal transducers; second messengers act on many enzymes; kinases phosphorylate multiple targets. There is potentially even more complexity in the nucleus, where numerous transcription factors, governed by a variety of biochemical devices, set the rate at which each gene is read out. Ultimately, however, this intricate network must produce simple answers to simple questions for each cell: Should the cell grow or not grow? Live or die? Progress toward a more differentiated state or remain as it is?

As we will see in the next chapter, there is an important purpose behind the extraordinary detail and duplicate function of these circuits. They are designed so that single disruptions here or there do not create malignant growth. A cell divides without restraint only when its circuitry has been disrupted at a number of key points: multiple mutations are required. Despite the many genetic insults sustained by a cell during its lifetime, this grand design ensures that transformation to cancer occurs only rarely.

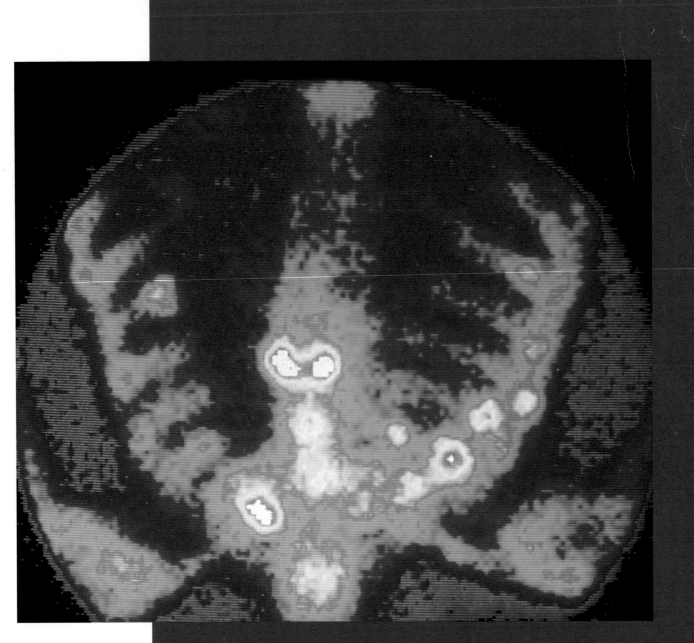

A radioisotope scan reveals a late stage of multistep
tumor progression in which a primary tumor has
spread to a number of sites in the rib cage,
yielding the metastases seen here as hot-spots on a
blue background.

7

MULTISTEP CARCINOGENESIS

T he transformation of normal cells into malignant cells involves many changes, since cancer cells differ from their normal counterparts in shape, dependence upon growth-stimulatory factors, metabolism of nutrients, and a host of other biochemical functions. How are so many changes in cell phenotype generated? Do they arise simultaneously as the result of a massive, coordinated shift in many cell functions? Or do they accumulate gradually through a series of successive alterations in the cell, each contributing some of the attributes that in sum constitute the malignant state?

A diverse set of observations, taken together, argues persuasively that the development of cancer depends upon a long and complex succession of changes in the behavior of a cell population. Each step enables precancerous cells to acquire some of the traits that together create the malignant growth of cancer cells.

INSIGHTS FROM EPIDEMIOLOGY

Cancer epidemiology provides a compelling though indirect demonstration that human cancer development is a multistep process. By surveying cancer incidence in large populations, epidemiologists gauge the chances that a person of a given age will develop a particular type of tumor. These age-dependent cancer risks yield important insights into the complex process of tumor formation.

Simple arithmetic can be used to interpret these cancer statistics. Assume that the occurrence of a tumor depends upon a single event or accident in the body and that the probability of such an event is similar from one year to the next; cancer risk should then increase in direct proportion to the number of years of elapsed lifetime—a 70-year-old should have a sevenfold greater chance of developing a colon carcinoma than a 10-year-old.

On the other hand, suppose that cancer depends upon the convergence of two rare accidents in the body, each occurring with a low but comparable probability during each year of life. We would then calculate cancer risk by multiplying the probability of one event by the probability of the other. Cancer risk would be proportional to the square of elapsed time (t^2), and the 70-year-old would

demonstrate a 49-fold greater risk than the 10-year-old.

In reality, however, we know that a 70-year-old man's risk of being diagnosed with

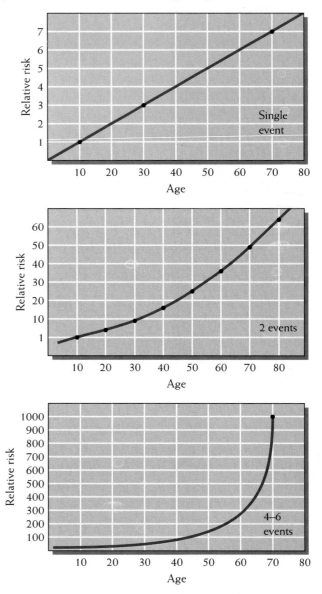

Predicted rates of colon cancer based on 1, 2, or 4–6 rate-limiting events.

colon cancer is more than 1000 times higher than that of a 10-year-old boy. Some statisticians maintain that the risk increases approximately as the fifth power of elapsed time (t^5), which implies a succession of *five* distinct events, each necessary in the progression toward colon cancer and each occurring with comparable probability per year. Whether these events must occur in a defined order or simply happen randomly is not made clear by this arithmetical analysis.

These data verify that colon cancer is a disease of people who have lived long enough to have experienced this complex succession of events, as revealed dramatically by curves plotting cancer incidence. Since each event is a rare accident, requiring years to occur, the whole process takes decades, an entire adult life span or longer; most of us will die from other causes before this sequence of events can reach its conclusion. But unusual exposure to carcinogens or inheritance of a cancer susceptibility gene presumably speeds up or leapfrogs over one or more of these steps, greatly increasing the likelihood of developing cancer during a normal life span.

Similar graphs of age-dependent cancer incidence, plotted for many other adult tumors, confirm multistep carcinogenesis. But no such analysis suggests the nature of the milestones along the road to malignancy. To learn that, we must examine the biology of cancer cells and cancerous growths. Can the multiple steps of tumor formation be described in concrete terms as discrete stopping points on the path from normality to malignancy? Are there cells or growths that are neither fully normal nor fully malignant?

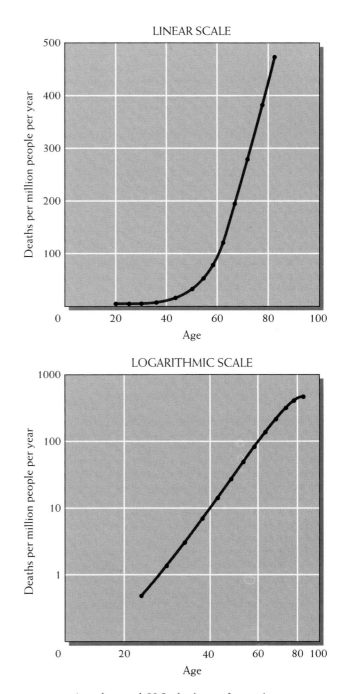

Actual annual U.S. death rate from colon cancer in relation to age, 1986.

Let us examine the various aberrant growths in the human colon, including several types of polyps (adenomas) and carcinomas. Do these tissues represent intermediate steps in tumor development? Are they related to one another, and if so, how?

MODELS OF CANCER FORMATION: THE COLON

Observations of aberrant growths in the colon are compatible with at least three different models of cancer formation. These models all assume that the unit of change is the individual colonic cell and its descendants and that the peculiarities of various normal and abnormal tissues are direct reflections of the traits of the individual cells that form them.

In the first model, the various types of colon growths represent an orderly sequence of changes through which a cell and its lineal descendants must pass to proceed from normality to malignancy. The second model, equally plausible, holds that a fully normal colon epithelial cell can undergo several possible changes: one path might allow the cell to proliferate into a polyp; a second might convert it directly into a carcinomatous cell capable of growing into a localized tumor; a third might transform the cell at once from fully normal to an aggressively growing cancer cell with the power to metastasize. Finally, a hybrid of these two models asserts that a normal colon cell may convert into several types of preneoplastic growths, some of which eventually lead to cancer, while others rarely or never do so.

The adenomas, thought to be intermediates between normal and malignant colon tissue, come in three varieties: tubular (glandular), tubulovillous, and villous. Each of these is seen in a variety of shapes and sizes. Tubular adenomas, frequently found in individuals over the age of 60, often form stalklike structures; their cells show tubules and secretory capacity but are otherwise not well differentiated. Villous adenomas look similar to the naked eye, but under a microscope they show fingerlike protrusions covered with very atypical cells. A tubulovillous adenoma has both tubular and villous structures in equal proportion.

Pathologists believe that one-quarter to one-half of villous adenomas carry within them islands of carcinoma cells, while tubular adenomas rarely do. The more villous a tubulovillous adenoma is, the larger its overall size—a measure that also correlates with the presence of carcinoma cells. Hyperplastic polyps seem never to contain carcinoma cells; adenomas less than 1.5 centimeters in diameter rarely do so; while 10 percent of the 1.5-centimeter adenomas and 45 percent of larger adenomas contain them.

The first scheme of colon tumorigenesis shown on the next page encompasses all this information, though it is not unambiguously proven. In this sequence, adenomas are the necessary precursors of carcinomas; some cells in a polyp evolve to a malignant growth state, spawning a carcinoma. (In reality, close physical proximity between an adenoma and a full-fledged carcinoma is seen in tissue only occasionally, presumably because the carcinomas rapidly overgrow and obliterate the polyps in which they arose.)

Other pathologists believe that villous adenomas become malignant three times more often than tubular growths. They might argue for the third scheme shown below.

Both models agree that carcinomas arise from polyp precursors, a notion reinforced by observations that specific, rare mutations detected in the DNA of some carcinomas can be found identically in the DNA of adjacent polyps. For example, some colon carcinomas carry the same point mutation in a K-ras gene as seen in a nearby polyp. The probability of such a genetic change occurring twice, independently, is extremely low; it is much more likely that this rare point mutation occurred only once in an ancestor of the polyp's cells, was perpetuated in all the growing polyp's descendant cells, and was inherited by carcinoma cells that arose directly or indirectly from a cell in the polyp. Very similar schemes of multistep tumor progression have been proposed for the bladder, cervix, and breast.

A CONFIRMING PHENOMENON

A familial colon cancer syndrome—adenomatous polyposis coli (APC)—provides another strong indication that benign polyps are the precursors of aggressive carcinomas. Individuals carrying the APC allele are predisposed to develop tubular polyps along the length of the colon. Up to a thousand of these polyps are often present without any obvious symptoms, but the individual affected develops colon carcinoma with almost 100 percent probability, often at several independent sites.

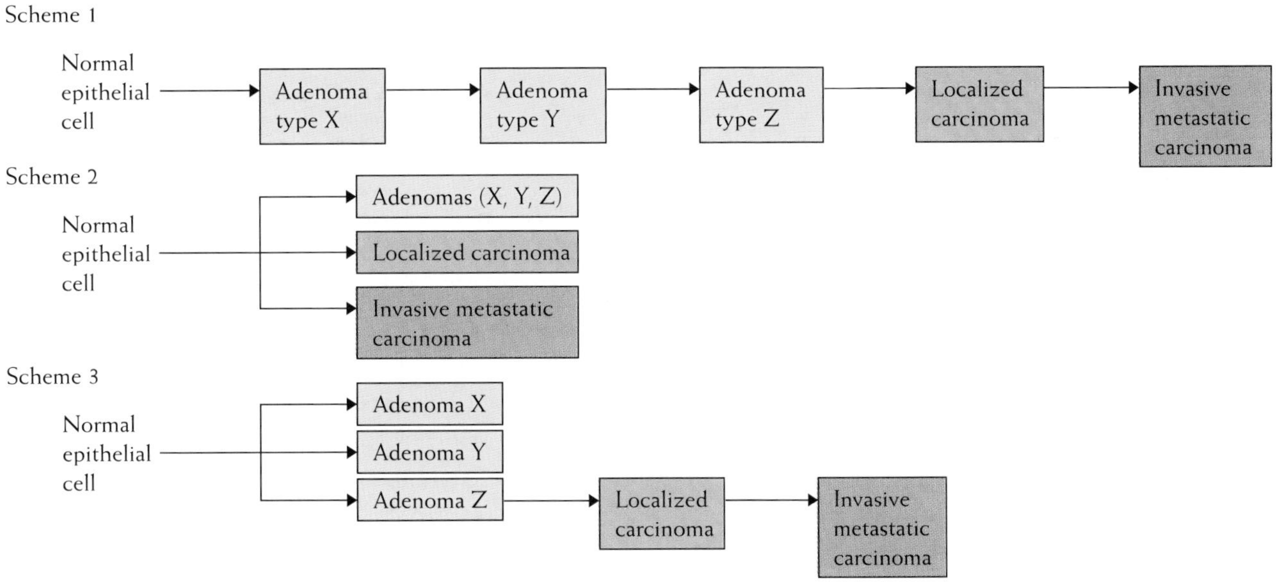

Three models of cancer formation in the colon.

These facts are explained most simply by a model in which (1) the APC allele predisposes not to cancer itself but to the development of many tubular polyps; (2) polyps are the obligatory precursors of carcinomas; (3) any single polyp has a low but finite chance of progressing to a carcinoma; and (4) the more polyps in the gut, the greater an individual's risk of developing a carcinoma. This association between polyps and increased risk of malignancy is so persuasive that individual polyps detected through colonoscopy in otherwise normal patients are surgically excised to preempt the development of a carcinoma; in individuals with familial polyposis, the entire colon is often removed as a preventive measure.

While provocative, all this leaves us with substantial uncertainty. In familial polyposis, 12 years on average elapse between the initial detection of widespread polyps and the first diagnosable cancer. What processes intervene during this time? Only a limited amount can be learned about these changes unless we observe them as they are happening. Since we cannot do this in human beings, we must turn to experimental animals.

MODELS OF CANCER FORMATION: MOUSE SKIN TUMORS

Some of the uncertainties left by clinical data can be addressed directly by animal models of cancer, where scientists can manipulate cell changes in target tissue, thereby affecting the site, rate, and extent of tumor development. Moreover, animal models allow us to study

individual steps in tumor formation while they occur rather than retrospectively years later. Here the relationships between benign and malignant growths can be defined much more precisely.

The most widely studied model of animal tumor induction involves the application of carcinogenic compounds to the skin on the back of a mouse. Mice treated following a specific experimental protocol develop skin carcinomas with high frequency and on a predictable schedule. The chemicals used to induce tumors can be applied directly to the target organ, in contrast to experimentally induced tumors of internal organs where the carcinogens often reach their targets through long and circuitous routes. In skin carcinogenesis, moreover, the experimenter can monitor the development of premalignant or malignant growths without the need to expose the affected organ surgically.

INITIATORS AND PROMOTERS

As first shown by Isaac Berenblum in 1941, skin tumor induction requires the application of two types of chemical compounds, termed initiators and promoters. A single application of the initiator 3-methyl-cholanthrene (3-MC), a compound isolated from coal tar, to a patch of mouse skin creates little if any change in its appearance. The treated area will remain normal for the life of the mouse if it is not further disturbed. Yet it appears that a number of cells in the treated area are altered irreversibly by exposure to the initiating chemical. This be-

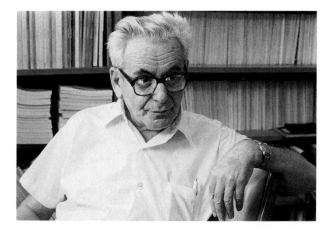

Isaac Berenblum.

comes obvious when the same patch of skin is then exposed to a promoting agent, such as tetradecanoyl phorbol acetate (TPA), a skin irritant extracted from the leaves of the croton plant. Repeated swabbing of the initiator-treated skin patch with TPA results in the appearance of benign, wartlike growths termed papillomas that have some similarities to adenomatous polyps in the gut; applying TPA to previously untreated skin patches fails to induce papillomas.

Target cells in mouse skin seem to require two types of stimuli to form papillomas. The initiator and promoter work together in a fixed sequence to induce these growths. The initiator creates a stable change in a small number of skin cells that enables them to respond to promoter treatment as long as a year after a single exposure to the initiating compound. They are, in effect, marked by the initiator, yet this mark is unapparent and initiated cells continue to participate in normal skin formation unless challenged by promoter treatment.

The great stability of the marking suggests that some genetic change is created in the initiator-treated cells and inherited by their descendants for many generations. In fact, initiating chemicals are invariably mutagenic when tested by the Ames assay (see Chapter 3). Conversely, promoting agents are poorly mutagenic, if at all. Reversing the order of initiator and promoter treatment fails to induce tumors, indicating the important differences in their roles.

Although promoting compounds like TPA have little or no mutagenic activity, they can act as strong growth stimulators, switching on a cell's growth-regulating circuits without directly damaging its genes. (See illustration on page 162 and detailed discussion on page 166.) In mouse skin, TPA's stimulatory action appears to be especially effective in forcing initiated cells to grow while leaving uninitiated cells unaffected. When the repeated treatment of initiated skin with promoter is stopped, the induced papillomas usually shrink and disappear.

If a promoter is applied often enough over a period of many months, some of the papillomas will eventually develop into malignant carcinomas. These carcinomas then take on their own dynamic, no longer requiring repeated stimulation by a promoter to survive and grow. In this respect they have become autonomous —unlike the papillomas, which will regress if deprived of continual stimulation by a promoter. Such acquired independence is the hallmark of cancer—it signals the development of a growth state that is governed by the tumor cells themselves and not by external factors such as promoters or other cells in the tissue.

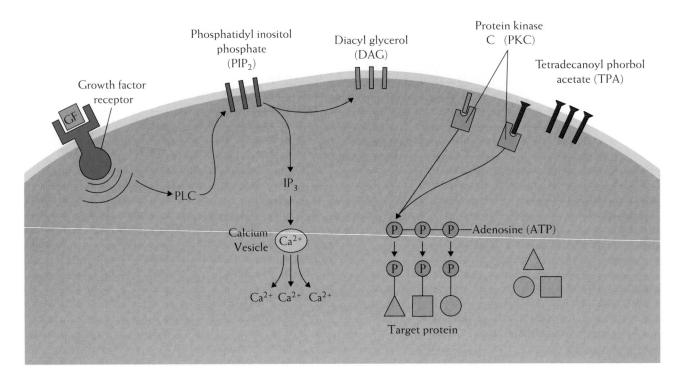

The tumor promoter TPA acts by mimicking a normal cellular second messenger, diacyl glycerol (DAG). In the normal cell, a growth factor causes its receptor to send out multiple signals inside the cell. One activates the enzyme phospholipase C (PLC), which then cleaves phosphatidyl inositol diphosphate (PIP$_2$) into DAG and inositol triphosphate (ITP). DAG then activates protein kinase C (PKC), which phosphorylates target proteins that in turn trigger growth. This complex process is short-circuited when an experimenter adds TPA, which binds to and directly activates PKC.

The conversion of papilloma to carcinoma cells, which occurs spontaneously at a low rate, is accelerated greatly by applying mutagenic agents to the papilloma. This suggests that there are at least two critical steps that depend upon damage to cellular genes: initiation, and the much later conversion of papilloma to carcinoma, which is often termed progression.

PROGRESSION AND DOUBLE MUTATION

Observations like these have inspired a simple scheme of how mouse skin carcinomas arise. First, an initiator enters many skin cells, damaging genes randomly. In a few cells, the initiating compound alters a critical growth-controlling gene; these cells, which become

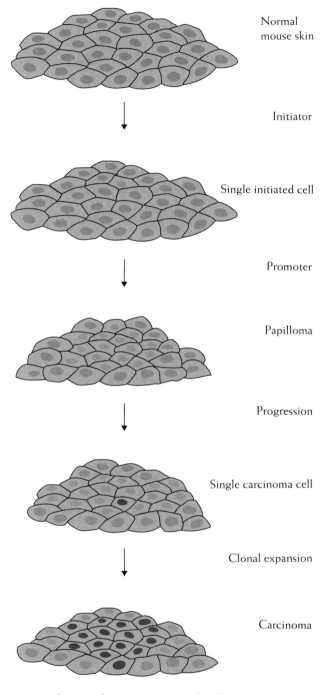

Normal mouse skin

↓

Initiator

Single initiated cell

↓

Promoter

Papilloma

↓

Progression

Single carcinoma cell

↓

Clonal expansion

Carcinoma

Process of tumorigenesis in induced mouse skin tumors.

initiated, may represent only one in every million skin cells and will remain inapparent amid their normal neighbors.

In the second phase of tumor formation, a promoting agent stimulates these few initiated cells to proliferate repeatedly until their descendants form visible papillomas, each made up of many millions of cells. In the third step, a mutagenic chemical is applied to the papilloma, damaging genes in many of its cells. As before, the mutagen acts with such randomness that only a minute proportion of papilloma cells—perhaps only one in a million—acquires a mutation that gives it further growth advantage. This rare papilloma cell is now doubly mutated, having acquired the first growth-promoting mutation from its initiated ancestor and a second during this later mutagenesis. This second genetic change allows the cell to proliferate without further promoter stimulus. Driven by these two distinct growth-promoting mutations, the skin cell and its descendants multiply rapidly to spawn a carcinoma.

CELL NUMBERS AND MALIGNANT PROGRESSION

Because the requisite second mutation (like all mutations) is a rare event, occurring only once in a million cells or so, a large population of papilloma cells is needed to produce a doubly mutated cell. This suggests that one important role of the promoter is to expand the population of initiated cells. The promoter need not be an exotic chemical like TPA, first used by

Direct and Indirect Tumor Promotion

Estrogens and hepatitis B virus, both tumor promoters that stimulate cell proliferation, act by fundamentally different mechanisms. Estrogens periodically direct healthy epithelial cells in the breast to proliferate beyond a basal level, creating a temporary hyperplasia. Hepatitis B virus stimulates liver cell proliferation indirectly; by killing infected cells, it prompts healthy cells to divide to make up for the loss. A wide variety of viral and chemical agents appear to act as indirect growth stimulators and as tumor promoters solely because their toxicity, killing some cells, forces compensatory proliferation of survivors within a damaged tissue. As with virtually all toxins, however, to be lethal they require a certain threshold concentration below which they are likely to be innocuous.

These facts enormously complicate the interpretation of many laboratory tests that depend upon introducing toxic (but possibly nonmutagenic) compounds into animals, usually rodents. These tests take one to two years and are expensive, so standard practice uses high doses of the test compound to increase the chance of significant numbers of tumors in a small cohort of animals within a short period of time. In fact, the highest tolerable doses are often used; beyond these levels, the animals sicken and die. As Bruce Ames (see Chapter 3) has pointed out, such compounds may induce cancer under these artificial conditions indirectly—toxic at very high doses, they kill cells, trigger compensatory proliferation, and in this way act as tumor promoters. At the far lower doses to which human beings are normally exposed, the same compounds may have no toxicity and thus no carcinogenicity whatsoever; that is, a thousandfold lower dose of such an agent may be a millionfold less carcinogenic. By this logic, it is foolish in many cases to extrapolate human risk from animal tests performed at maximum tolerated dose. One example is saccharin, which in enormously high doses is apparently toxic and carcinogenic for the rat-bladder epithelium but at the thousandfold lower doses normally encountered as a human food additive is apparently nontoxic and probably totally innocuous.

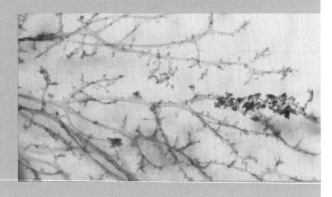

Developing network of milk ducts in the breast of a two-month-old mouse. The grapelike cluster (right) represents localized benign hyperproliferation of duct tissue, as might be seen in a transgenic, oncogene-bearing mouse before the onset of a mammary carcinoma.

Berenblum on mouse skin because of its known irritative powers. More common agents appear to achieve the same result in other organs. For example, the estrogen hormones released as part of the normal menstrual cycle seem to promote the development of mammary carcinomas, presumably because they stimulate growth of the epithelial cells in the milk ducts. As before, the promoter encourages the proliferation of cells in a specific target tissue, creating the large cell populations in which the rare genetic events needed to further the cancer process can occur.

The cell division induced by promoters is, we should note, intrinsically mutagenic, because the copying of chromosomal DNA during genome replication is prone to occasional errors, which create spontaneous mutations that can be as dangerous as those actively induced by external mutagens. Such mutagenesis, associated with normal cell division, seems to explain how tumor promoters can occasionally induce the progression of skin papillomas to carcinomas even without the application of a mutagenic carcinogen. By forcing cell division, the promoter causes cells to accumulate mutations, albeit not as rapidly as they would in response to an actively mutagenic chemical.

The connection between stimulating cell growth and promoting cancer is confirmed by the study of carcinogenesis in other organs. The chronic inflammation and associated cell proliferation seen in ulcerative colitis favor development of colon cancer. Analogously, frequent alcohol consumption acts as an irritant in the epithelial lining of the esophagus, killing cells that must be replaced; the resulting proliferation again seems to favor the development of esophageal cancer.

ONCOGENES AND INITIATION

Fascinating genetic and biochemical details have emerged about the molecular processes underlying mouse skin carcinogenesis. We now know the identity of the elusive target altered during initiation: skin tumors initiated by 3-MC usually carry copies of a Ha-ras gene that has been mutated at its twelfth codon. When the resulting mutant ras allele is isolated from these cells by gene cloning and introduced into NIH3T3 cells, it acts as a potent transforming oncogene, as described in Chapter 4. The fact that dozens of independently induced skin tumors carry the identical Ha-ras mutation raises another question: How can 3-MC molecules, which strike randomly at DNA, almost invariably create the same mutation in the twelfth codon of the ras gene?

The answer seems to derive from the nature of most mutations in carcinogen-treated cells, the vast majority of which are either deleterious or neutral (evoking no obvious changes in cell behavior). On very rare occasions, the carcinogen affects a gene sequence whose alteration confers active growth advantage on the cell, which now outcompetes all others in the tissue, growing into the large clone of descendants that make up a tumor. There may be, in fact, only a small number of sites in the genome where point mutations (the sort created by 3-MC) result in growth-favoring alleles. The ras genes are known to contain several of these target sequences.

Here is an experiment suggesting that the observed ras mutation is essential, indeed sufficient, to initiate a skin tumor. Harvey sarcoma virus, which carries an oncogenic allele of the

Ha-ras gene (and gave this oncogene its name), can be used to infect normal mouse skin, which then behaves as if it had been treated by the initiating compound 3-MC: when subsequently exposed to a tumor promoter like TPA, it forms papillomas. This result is striking proof that the activities of an initiator can be mimicked entirely by inserting a ras oncogene into skin cells. Any other effects of the initiator seem to be irrelevant.

PROMOTION AND PROGRESSION

How does the promoter contribute to cancer formation? Work over the past decade has shown that TPA has only one molecular target in the cell: it binds to protein kinase C, a serine–threonine kinase in the cytoplasm. This enzyme, once activated by TPA, attaches phosphate groups to serine and threonine amino acid residues of other target proteins in the cell, whose functions are altered thereby. (See the illustration on page 162.)

We know from the previous chapter that protein kinase C (PKC) is a central regulator of cell growth. The TPA molecules that bind to PKC and activate it are foreign, introduced by the experimenter into the normal skin cell. But TPA is effectively mimicking a natural intracellular compound—diacylglycerol—that the cell normally produces in response to external growth-stimulatory signals such as growth factors. In this way TPA can insinuate itself into a cell's growth-regulating circuitry, turn on a critical switch, and activate a variety of cellular responses.

Even the mystery of how mouse skin cells progress from forming papillomas to forming carcinomas has been solved at the molecular level, 50 years after the process of tumor progression was first described. Mouse skin carcinoma cells all carry mutations in their p53 tumor suppressor genes (see Chapter 5), in addition to the ras oncogene mutation already present in their papillomatous ancestors. Why then does it require two (or more) mutant genes to create a cancer cell? How can we understand these two mutations and their interactions? The complex tissue of a mouse skin does not yield the answer readily.

CARCINOGENESIS BY A SINGLE ONCOGENE?

A powerful approach to this question was suggested by the Ha-ras oncogene experiment. Rather than wait for a carcinogen to activate a cellular proto-oncogene, a researcher can introduce an already mutated oncogene by infecting a cell with a tumor virus or by introducing DNA clones of the oncogene directly into cells—a process called transfection.

As discussed earlier, transfection of a ras oncogene into NIH3T3 cells converts them into tumor cells. But this result is complicated by the fact that the NIH3T3 cells are aberrant even before they acquire the oncogene by transfection. Because they are immortalized—having the ability to multiply indefinitely in culture—these cells already exhibit a trait typical of cancer cells.

How would a completely normal cell respond to an introduced oncogene? Normal cells from rat or mouse embryo tissues also can be grown in culture. These cells, largely fibro-

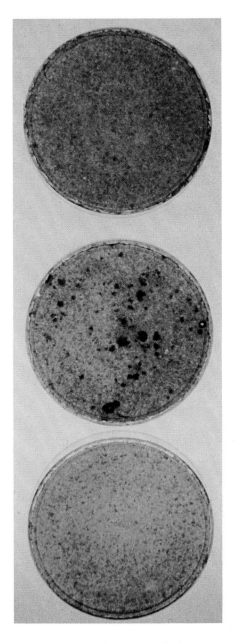

Rat embryo fibroblasts into which a ras oncogene (top), a myc oncogene (bottom), or both oncogenes (center) have been introduced by gene transfer (transfection). Only the two oncogenes together induce foci of transformed cells.

Pairs of Collaborating Oncogenes

ras, ros, src, yes, sea, erbB, or fps	myc
ras	N-myc
ras	L-myc
ras	Adenovirus E1A
Polyoma/middle-T antigen	Polyomavirus large-T antigen
ras	SV40 large-T antigen
ras	Papillomavirus E7

An oncogene from the left column can collaborate with its counterpart from the right column to transform a fully normal rat embryo fibroblast into a sarcoma cell.

blasts, are not immortalized and represent good approximations of the cells found in healthy tissues in the intact animal.

Introducing cloned DNA carrying a powerful ras oncogene into rat embryo fibroblasts had surprisingly little effect on their growth properties in culture; they still formed normal monolayers. Failing to transform these embryo cells with a ras oncogene, experimenters tried the myc oncogene frequently encountered in human tumors. Again, there was little effect on the cells' growth properties.

Both ras and myc oncogenes had been isolated previously from human tumor cells. Each apparently played an important role in inducing malignant behavior, yet neither was able to transform these normal rat embryo cells. We may conclude that truly normal fibroblastic cells cannot be converted into tumor cells by the action of a single oncogene (in this case, ras or myc). More changes are apparently needed.

ONCOGENE COLLABORATION

A simple experiment yielded the sought-after transformation. When the two oncogenes were transfected simultaneously into the embryo cells, thick, robust foci appeared and expanded aggressively in the petri dish. These cells showed the loss of contact inhibition and the rounded shape typical of cancer cells. Cells from these foci, inoculated into young rats, rapidly proliferated to form tumors; cells carrying only a single oncogene failed to do so. In short, this focus-forming assay, carried out in culture, is a good predictor of tumor-forming abilities in the living animal.

Cancer Viruses and Multistep Tumorigenesis

No virus implicated in causing human cancer acts as a complete carcinogen. Each only pushes an infected cell one or two steps along the road to malignancy; complete transformation seems to require the same random, somatic mutations that intervene in the formation of nonviral tumors. The human papillomavirus genomes implicated in initiating cervical carcinomas, for example, carry two genes (E6 and E7) whose products bind and apparently inactivate the cervical epithelial cell's p53 and Rb suppressor proteins, respectively (see Chapter 5). This binding is necessary (but perhaps not sufficient) for the outgrowth of benign cervical growths. Epstein-Barr virus, through the actions of its EBNA-2, EBNA-3A, EBNA-3C, LMP-1, and LMP-2 genes, immortalizes lymphocytes, a precondition creating a susceptibility, in malarial Africa, to Burkitt's lymphoma. Additional somatic mutations (for example, myc

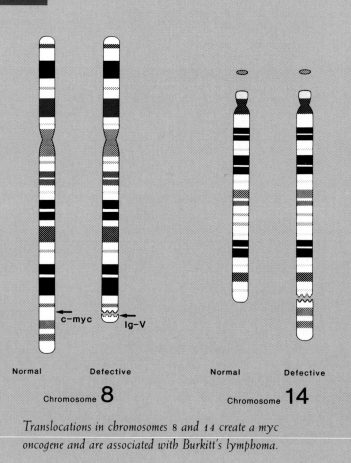

Translocations in chromosomes 8 and 14 create a myc oncogene and are associated with Burkitt's lymphoma.

On the basis of this experiment, we can conclude that oncogenes like ras and myc can cooperate to transform a normal cell into a malignant one; neither acting alone suffices (see the table on page 167 for other examples). Such collaboration can be explained by examining the biological changes induced by each oncogene. The ras oncogene causes changes in cell shape and allows cells to grow independently of anchorage to a solid substrate. The myc oncogene immortalizes cells, causing them to proliferate indefinitely. Both alterations appear necessary to produce an aggressively growing tumor cell. We conclude that each oncogene makes a unique contribution to cell transformation, and the actions of each complement those of the other.

Many other pairs of oncogenes have been found to collaborate in transforming cells. One of the genes that works with the ras oncogene is a mutant form of the p53 tumor suppressor gene; like myc, it is adept at immortalizing

translocations) must intervene to force the virus-infected cells beyond their pre-neoplastic state. Human T-cell lymphotropic virus (HTLV-I), acting through its tax gene, creates at worst a benign lymphocytic proliferation that may, after several decades, progress with low (1 to 5 percent) probability into a leukemia or lymphoma. The most common viral carcinogen worldwide, hepatitis B virus, apparently has no oncogenes at all. Its contribution to tumorigenesis seems to derive from the widespread liver damage it causes over many decades of chronic infection. The proliferation of liver cells to compensate for the continual virus-induced cell death seems to be critical for the development of genetic changes that ultimately lead to hepatocellular carcinoma. Many people infected with HBV as infants will develop tumors only in the sixth or seventh decade of life.

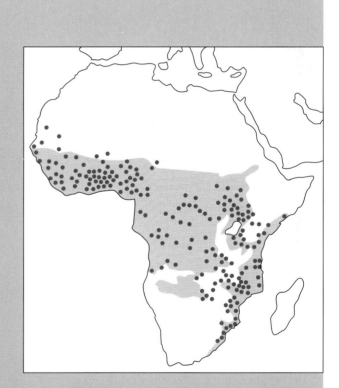

The distribution of malaria in Africa (shaded area), compared with the cases of Burkitt's lymphoma documented by Denis Burkitt in 1962 (dots)—a correlation that has yet to be fully explained.

Oncogene Collaboration in Various Cell Types

CELL TYPE	NUCLEAR[a] ONCOGENE	CYTOPLASMIC[a] ONCOGENE
Avian chondroblasts	myc	src
Avian macrophages	myc or myb	erbB, src, fps, mil Ha-ras, ros, yes, sea
Rat prostate cells	myc	ras
Splenocytes	myc	ras
Rat kidney	myc, E1A	ras
Mouse erythroid	myc	raf
Mouse myelocytes	myc	abl
Mouse B lymphocytes	myc	ras, raf
Rat adrenocortical	myc	ras, src
Chick neuroretina	myc	mil
Mouse pre-B	myc	bcl-2
Avian erythroblast	erbA	erbB
Avian fibroblasts	erbB	erbB
Avian macrophages	myc	mil

[a]The terms nuclear and cytoplasmic refer to the location of the oncogene products.

cells. We now know that many spontaneously immortalized cells, like the NIH3T3 cells described earlier, carry mutant alleles of p53 genes. These mutations explain both the spontaneous immortalization of these cells and their responsiveness to a ras oncogene introduced by transfection. They also explain the presence of the mutant forms of ras and p53 genes coexisting in the mouse skin tumors. As noted in Chapter 5, mutant alleles of the p53 gene are also found in more than half of malignant human tumors.

The phenomenon of oncogene cooperation teaches a number of important lessons about multistep carcinogenesis. It shows that the distinct genetic alterations creating each activated oncogene result in distinct effects on cell behavior. It suggests, moreover, that each step in the progression of a normal cell to a tumor cell may reflect the activation of a particular oncogene (or the inactivation of a suppressor gene like p53). It seems that a cell population must sustain a number of mutations in critical growth-controlling genes before it reaches malignancy. We now begin to understand why mouse skin cells require at least two (and perhaps more) mutations before they grow like truly autonomous cancer cells.

TRANSGENIC MODELS OF CANCER FORMATION: ONCOGENIC ACTIVITY

The use of embryo cells has allowed us to define the genetic elements that may contribute to cancer, but it has taken us away from tumor progression as it occurs in a living tissue. Although focus formation in a petri dish is often a good indicator of the ability of cells to form tumors in an animal, many of the complexities of cancer formation in a living tissue cannot even be approximated in culture. Thus, we need to return to the study of cell transformation in a live model, armed now with our ex-

tensive knowledge about oncogenes and their collaborative abilities. Recall that the introduction of chemical carcinogens into laboratory animals creates oncogenes in a target organ randomly and then only after many months of treatment, making this approach slow and imprecise. One solution is to reengineer the genome of a laboratory mouse so that specific oncogenes are expressed in specific tissues at predetermined times in the mouse's development. The genetic program of the mouse, rather than the random, uncontrollable actions of a mutation, is now the force activating oncogenes within cells.

This strategy involves the creation of transgenic mice, each genetically normal except that one or more novel genes, such as oncogenes, have been added experimentally to its genome. A DNA clone of the gene of interest, injected into a fertilized mouse egg, becomes linked to chromosomal DNA in the zygote and is subsequently inherited by cells of the resulting embryo. Since the transgene is also incorporated into the genome of gonadal cells (ovary and testis), it is thereby transmitted to succeeding generations of mice. In this way it becomes possible to create a unique mouse

Transgenic mice show dramatically the role of non-mutagenic tumor promoters. In one mouse strain, which expresses the H-ras oncogene in certain of its skin cells, young males develop multiple benign skin papillomas (shown), while young females do not; some of these papillomas eventually progress to malignant, invasive carcinomas. Several males placed in a single cage, moreover, display the most papillomas. Why are males so susceptible? The process is driven entirely by inter-male rivalry—frequent fights yield abrasions, and papillomas arise at the wound sites. The promoting agent here is tissue damage that, by triggering cell proliferation as part of the wound-healing process, acts synergistically with the ras oncogene to create these growths.

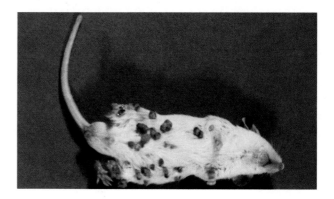

breed, all of whose members carry the novel transgene.

Separate experiments have, by now, inserted hundreds of distinct genes, including many oncogenes, into the germ lines of mice. Before injection, these genes can be custom designed so that they are turned on and expressed in only one specific mouse tissue. For example, a myc oncogene can be constructed that is expressed only in breast tissue; mammary carcinomas will then arise on a predictable timetable after the birth of the mouse.

In one of the first such experiments, mice carrying a myc oncogene designed to be expressed in breast tissue showed mammary carcinomas with high frequency beginning at 15 weeks of age; by 12 months, 60 percent show these tumors. Similarly, mice carrying an SV40 large-T oncogene engineered to be expressed in the insulin-producing cells produced pancreatic carcinomas three to four months after birth.

These and other transgenic animal strains hold enormous promise for cancer research. They allow scientists to study the stages of carcinogenesis in an organism in which cancer formation follows a well-defined timetable. In these mice, however, a single discrete genetic change represented by the introduced transgene appears to be sufficient to create a tumor—undermining the theory that multiple genetic changes are required.

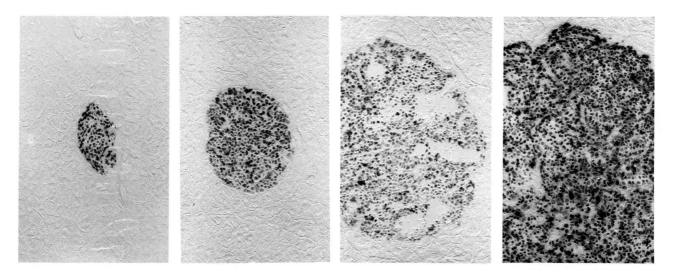

Tumor progression in an islet cell of a transgenic mouse engineered to express the large-T oncoprotein. Left: normal islet cell; second panel: hyperplastic islet; third panel: angiogenesis with several hemorrhages (clear areas); right: carcinoma.

CARCINOGENESIS BY A SINGLE TRANSGENE?

Appearances can be deceiving. By noting the precise times at which tumors appear, biologists recognized that the introduced transgene initiates the steps leading to cancer but cannot complete the process on its own. Consider, for example, the SV40 large-T transgenic mice that express this oncogene in the islet cells of the pancreas, the small islands of cells that make insulin. While all their pancreatic islets express the viral oncoprotein, only 50 to 70 percent develop hyperplasia (overgrowth) first apparent by four weeks of age. Of these hyperplastic islets, only 1 to 2 percent develop, within two months, into carcinomas. So although virtually all the cells in the target tissue may express the oncogenic transgene, only a few go on to produce an expanding population of progeny cells that ultimately progresses into a tumor. By this measure, the single oncogene is necessary for cancer development but not sufficient. It creates the early hyperplasia, but other, random events must occur later to push the process to completion—apparently somatic mutations occurring in a few of the many cells that are already expressing the oncogenic transgene.

These mutations presumably serve to activate oncogenes or inactivate tumor suppressor genes. One illustration of this comes from experiments in which mice carrying a transgenic oncogene are then infected with a murine leukemia virus (MLV). The virus infection hastens the appearance of tumors. The genomes of these tumors, when examined, are found to carry MLV proviruses that have activated proto-oncogenes by integrating next to them (insertional mutagenesis; see Chapter 4). These virus-activated oncogenes, which represent somatic mutational events, appear to collaborate with the inherited transgene to create the tumor, reminding us of the oncogene collaborations described earlier. For example, MLV-infected myc-transgenic mice often show tumors carrying a virus-activated pim-1 oncogene. Mouse genetics can also be used to make the point. If we breed ras-transgenic mice with myc-transgenic mice, the doubly transgenic offspring show tumors much more rapidly than their singly transgenic parents. We conclude, once again, that either of these transgenes alone does not suffice to create a full-fledged tumor.

TRANSGENIC MODELS OF CANCER FORMATION: TUMOR SUPPRESSION

Success in these transgenic mouse experiments proves what researchers have long taken for granted but never before shown directly: that oncogenes can cause cancer within a living tissue. In the absence of these experimental results, skeptics might have argued that the oncogenes isolated from human and animal tumors represent incidental consequences of cancer—side issues rather than central agents that cause disease.

But while clearly very useful, these transgenic models fall short in one significant respect. Tumorigenesis involves both the activation of oncogenes and the equally important inactivation of tumor suppressor genes, but transgenic mouse models represent only the part of the process involving oncogene activation. Modeling the steps involved in the loss of suppressor genes would seem to require a different technology, one to knock out genes already present in normal mouse DNA.

In fact such techniques, developed in recent years, are being used to create strains of mice carrying inactivated alleles of tumor suppressor genes like p53, Rb (retinoblastoma), NF-1 (neurofibromatosis), and WT-1 (Wilms' tumor). Mice have been developed that totally lack p53 gene function: both chromosomal copies of this suppressor gene have been inactivated. Perhaps surprisingly, these mice develop and are born normally, but three weeks after birth they begin to show tumors; by six months, all have succumbed to cancer. Mice lacking both copies of the Rb suppressor gene die in the womb five or six days before term. These experiments show that the p53 gene is not essential for normal embryonic development but is necessary to protect the newborn mouse against cancer, while the Rb gene is apparently needed for normal development in the womb, so that its role in cancer protection after birth cannot even be tested by this method. (The long-term cancer susceptibility of Rb heterozygous mice, normal at birth, is being studied by a number of research teams.) An ongoing project to create genetically altered mice that carry both activated oncogenes and inactivated suppressor genes will allow us to study in detail the respective contributions of these genes to cancer development.

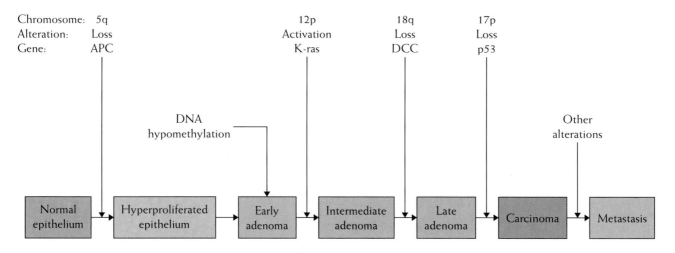

Genetic changes occurring during evolution of a typical colon carcinoma. These changes are only statistically associated with each step in tumor progression, and each tumor may take a slightly different path to the endpoint.

How Do Gene Changes Correlate with Stages of Human Tumor Growth?

A major goal of current cancer research is to associate each step in the formation of a human tumor with the alteration of a distinct, identifiable oncogene or tumor suppressor gene. This goal is far from realization. Activation of single oncogenes has been associated with certain specific stages of tumor formation in a variety of tissues, but the other contributory genetic changes in these tumors remain enigmatic.

In bone marrow, for instance, activation of the abl oncogene through chromosomal translocation seems to be a relatively early event in the process that leads to chronic myelogenous leukemia. Similarly, the premalignant cells of myelodysplastic syndrome often carry activated ras oncogenes. Disappointingly, the genes involved in subsequent steps are not yet known, though some acute myelogenous leukemia cells do acquire mutated p53 alleles.

Conversely, there are tumor types in which the later molecular steps have been identified but early ones remain elusive. In childhood neuroblastoma, for instance, amplification of the N-myc gene is correlated with late-stage aggressive growth and resistance to therapy. (Gene amplification, as we have noted earlier, causes genes to accumulate in many copies per cell, rather than the usual two.) Similarly, in human mammary and ovarian carcinomas, amplification of both the erb B-1 and the erb B-2 (neu) oncogenes suggests a poor clinical prognosis, since tumor cells carrying these abnor-

malities often metastasize. Association of these amplifications with late developments in tumor progression is probably more than incidental; indeed, it is likely that these gene amplifications actually drive the tumor cells into more aggressive growth.

A Model of Correlation: The Colon

Human colon cancer has provided the clearest picture to date of how discrete genetic changes correlate with specific steps in the development of a tumor. Individuals suffering from familial adenomatous polyposis (FAP) carry alterations in the APC (adenomatous polyposis coli) gene that trigger formation of up to a thousand colonic polyps. This APC gene, which also seems to be altered by somatic mutations in nonfamilial (sporadic) tumors, acts at the very earliest stages of colon carcinogenesis.

Recent evidence has shown that up to half of the tubular polyps carry activated K-ras oncogenes in their DNA. Many of the larger, villous adenomas not only carry these ras oncogenes but also show losses in their DCC tumor suppressor gene copies. Later in the process, full carcinomas carry mutations of their p53 suppressor genes. For the first time we see, in a single type of cancer, a relationship between defined stages of tumor progression and multiple, specific gene alterations. This sequence of events is not invariable, however, and may differ in some colon cancers.

These correlations are consistent with a model in which each stage reached by an evolving tumor cell population is triggered by the activation of an oncogene or the inactivation of a suppressor gene. Moreover, in many colon carcinoma cells a mutant ras oncogene coexists with a mutant allele of p53; recall that these same genes can collaborate to transform embryo cells in culture.

A PARADOX

Beyond changes in the oncogenes and tumor suppressor genes, other types of genes still to be discovered must play equally important roles in removing normal controls on cell growth. The involvement of a totally different type of gene, for example, is suggested by a paradox not easily resolved by current models. Certain tumor cells contain changes at up to 12 different sites in the genome. A well-documented example comes from small-cell lung carcinoma (SCLC), a tumor common in heavy cigarette smokers: almost all SCLC tumors appear to have changes in both Rb gene copies, both p53 genes, and a still unidentified gene on the short arm of chromosome 3. In addition, they often show amplification of the myc gene or one of the myc-like genes (N-myc or L-myc).

Each of these genetic changes is a low-probability event, occurring once in a thousand (10^{-3}) to (more typically) once in a million (10^{-6}) times per cell generation. The likelihood of all the events occurring together—the product of all the probabilities—would seem to be extraordinarily small, perhaps once in 10^{30} or more cell divisions. The 10 to 30 years that

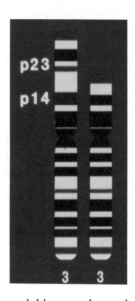

An interstitial deletion in the p23 band of chromosome 3 seen in some small-cell lung carcinomas. This suggests loss of a tumor suppressor gene, one of many changes occurring during tumor formation.

it actually takes such tumors to develop seem far too short a time to accommodate this highly improbable series of events. How can a cell genome change in so many ways, within such a limited period?

One answer has come from reexamining the mutation rates used in these calculations. In recent years, researchers who measured mutation rates in normal and tumor cells found that the latter often show dramatically increased mutation rates per cell generation. One tumor cell line, for example, increased by at least 10,000-fold the tendency to amplify its genes. Such amplification is one aspect of genomic instability that may be typical of many cancer cells.

This finding suggests that the cellular machinery designed to maintain the proper number and configuration of genes often breaks down in tumor cells. The increased mutation rates that result may lead to the rapid accumulation of large numbers of aberrant genes, which would greatly accelerate the genetic evolution of the tumor cell population as a whole. In effect, cancer cells may acquire a highly mutable, plastic genome during their progression to malignancy.

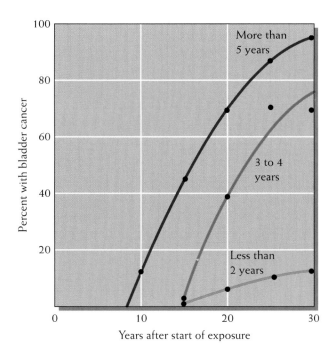

Timing of appearance of bladder cancer in a group of 78 men exposed to 2-naphthylamine (divided into three groups, according to total duration of exposure). Long-time exposure favors mutations in multiple genes, thereby accelerating multistep carcinogenesis.

HEREDITARY CANCER SYNDROMES

This notion of increased mutability provides insight into the origin of certain kinds of unusual inherited syndromes, including Bloom's syndrome, Fanconi's anemia, ataxia telangiectasia, and xeroderma pigmentosum. In each of these syndromes, there is evidence of a congenital defect in the DNA repair mechanisms that cells throughout the body rely upon to erase and repair errors caused either by external mutagenic agents—such as chemicals, X rays, and ultraviolet (UV) radiation—or by their own accidental miscopying of genomic DNA. Individuals whose cells carry one of these repair defects suffer the same numbers of DNA-damaging events as the rest of us but are unable to repair the damage. Consequently, the heavy burden of mutations that accumulate in the cellular DNA of these patients, ranging from point mutations to large-scale changes in chromosome structure, results in unusually high rates of certain malignancies.

One well-known example is provided by xeroderma pigmentosum patients, who must avoid all direct sunlight lest its UV rays create widespread genetic damage in skin cells, generating skin carcinomas and melanomas. In these people, the increased mutation rates do not occur because of deterioration of the DNA repair apparatus during tumor evolution; rather, this defect affects all their cells long before tumorigenesis begins. The course of tumor progression is accelerated, thereby increasing cancer rates in these patients.

Mutation beyond Carcinogenesis: Evading the Body's Defenses

Our descriptions of multistep tumorigenesis have been built around the notion that developing tumor cells acquire an ever-increasing growth advantage through gene mutations. These mutations create genetic variability; the cells with the most growth-favoring mutations proliferate rapidly, outcompete normal cells, and soon dominate. But for a tumor cell to survive and compete successfully in the complex environment of the living body, it must do more than proliferate. A tumor must defeat the host's defenses and become an effective parasite. Accomplishing this may depend upon its abilities to evade immune surveillance, to metastasize, and to attract a blood supply.

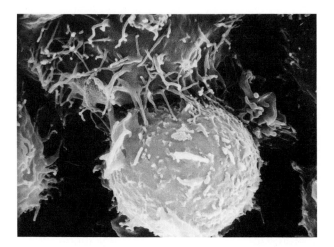

A killer T cell makes contact with a smaller tumor cell.

The importance of immune defenses against cancer remains a matter of great controversy. One school of thought argues that specialized cells of the immune system continuously survey tissues for small nests of tumor cells that, once recognized, are attacked and wiped out. This view is supported by the discovery of natural killer (NK) lymphocytes that seem able to identify and destroy many types of tumor cells. If immune surveillance by these and other cell types is indeed important in antitumor defenses, then cancer cells must acquire an ability to elude the immune system.

One strategy for evasion may derive from the mechanism that certain immune cells use to recognize tumor cells. Tumor cells may display specific antigens on their surfaces that alert the immune system to their presence. All cells display class I histocompatibility antigens on their surfaces, but N-myc oncogene amplification in advanced childhood neuroblastomas causes the tumor cells to decrease expression of these class I antigens drastically—perhaps enabling the neuroblastoma cells to evade detection by becoming antigenically invisible to the immune cells responsible for recognizing and killing tumor cells.

Mutation beyond Carcinogenesis: Obtaining a Blood Supply

Another issue is nourishment of the developing tumor. Having escaped the immune system, incipient tumors must secure an adequate blood supply to ensure growth. Without vascularization—small arteries, capillaries, and veins—the tumor cannot acquire nutrients and oxygen and eliminate wastes like carbon dioxide and lactic acid. Tumors more than a few millimeters in diameter soon stop growing unless they have access to circulating blood.

Access to the blood supply requires the growth of new vessels that must invade the tumor from adjacent normal tissue. This process is termed angiogenesis. Tumors develop the ability to release specific growth factors— angiogenic factors—that induce blood vessels to penetrate the tumor mass. As an illustration of angiogenesis, tumor cells taken from an advanced, aggressive tumor and implanted into the cornea of a rabbit quickly induce dramatic

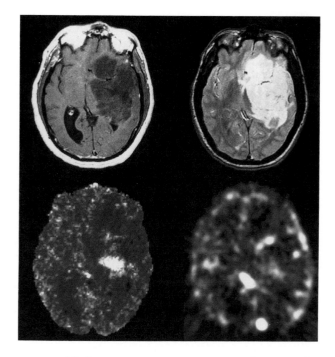

Nuclear magnetic resonance imaging (MRI) renders images of a tumor as it grows inside the patient. The top left image reveals a slowly growing malignant brain tumor—a low-grade glioma (large dark area on right). A refinement of the technique allows the volume of the blood flow to be visualized (lower left). The tumor appears heterogeneous and poorly vascularized (dark areas) except for one small patch (bright spot). This group of cells, over eight years, proceeded to expand into an aggressive, ultimately lethal tumor (right images).

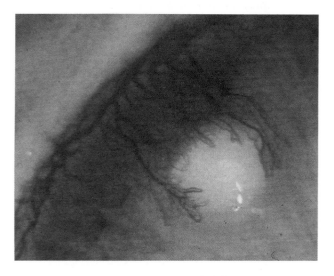

Tumor extract partially purified for angiogenic activity in a sustained-release polymer implanted in the rabbit cornea. The new capillaries have grown around it, being attracted by fibroblast growth factor present in the extract.

ingrowth of a large array of capillaries from nearby vessels. Injection into the cornea of fibroblast growth factor (FGF), a known angiogenic factor, mimics this recruitment of a vessel network. Angiogenesis is clearly a critical step in tumor progression, and in some well-studied tumors this vessel-building clearly accompanies—and may trigger—the conversion of relatively benign to more malignant growths.

A striking example derives from a study of human breast cancer patients who had either localized small tumors or tumors with aggressive metastatic spread. The density of blood vessels was measured in tumor samples taken from the patients' breasts. Women who had poorly vascularized tumors (0 to 33 microvessels per microscope field) were found to have a low rate of metastasis. Those whose local tumors had attracted many vessels (more than 100 per field) showed distant metastases. These latter tumor cells gained the ability to grow both locally and distantly by rapidly recruiting blood vessels to nourish them. For many types of tumors, the ability to become vascularized may be a prerequisite to metastatic spread.

MUTATION BEYOND CARCINOGENESIS: METASTASIS

Metastasis usually occurs as a late manifestation of tumor development. Recall that in human cancer, tumor cells that seed in distant sites throughout the body (metastases) are responsible for more than 90 percent of patient deaths; primary tumors kill only rarely. The process of metastasis, poorly understood, is composed of several discrete steps.

In epithelial tumors, the cancer cell must invade through the basement membrane that underlies the normal epithelium. Once the tumor has gained a foothold in the connective

tissue that underlies the basement membrane, clumps of tumor cells may break off from the primary mass, invading nearby blood or lymphatic vessels (intravasation). These vessels may then carry tumor cells to distant sites in the circulatory or lymphatic systems, where they can become trapped. By leaving the vessels (extravasation), these cells may then colonize a tissue very different from the one in which they originated: breast carcinomas often metastasize to bone, melanomas to the lungs and brain, and colon carcinomas to the liver.

Each of these steps represents complex biochemical interactions between the tumor cell and its environment. The nature of the genetic changes that enable tumor cells to execute these steps is unclear. Oncogenes may play a role, but unrelated types of genes and associated biological processes may be even more important. For instance, tumor cells often se-

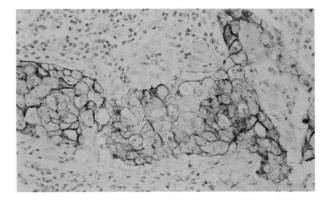

In this slide of a lymph node from a breast-cancer patient, antibodies against metalloproteinases cause metastatic cancer cells to stain brown. These proteinases, released by the cancer cell, degrade the extracellular matrix, allowing invasive metastasis to nearby tissue sites.

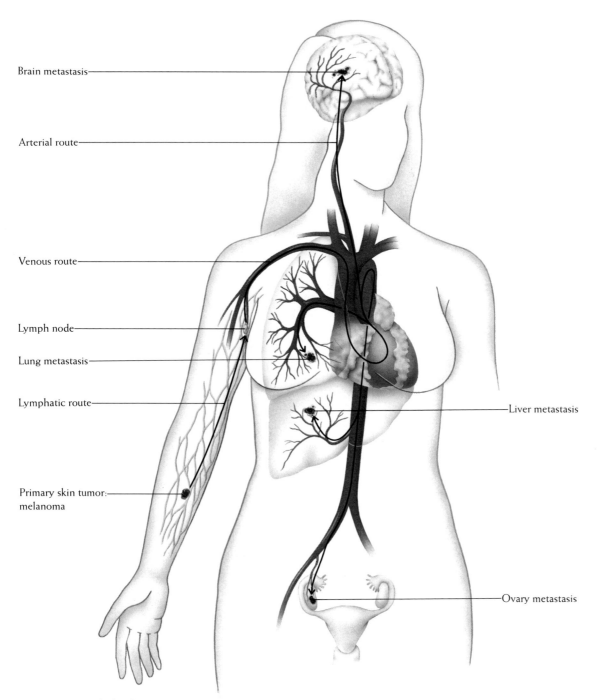

Brain metastasis

Arterial route

Venous route

Lymph node

Lung metastasis

Lymphatic route

Primary skin tumor:
melanoma

Liver metastasis

Ovary metastasis

Metastatic spread of malignant melanoma can begin when cells from a tumor on, for example, the forearm invade a lymphatic vessel and are carried to a node. Entering a blood vessel, the cells can be carried through the heart to other parts of the body—the brain, the lungs, the liver, or the ovaries.

crete enzymes called proteases into the extra-cellular space, which break down and destroy the matrix of connective protein molecules around the cell. Carcinoma cells, for example, release collagenases that dissolve the collagen that surrounds, anchors, and immobilizes cells within a tissue and forms the skeleton of the basement membrane through which metastasiz-ing carcinoma cells invade. By degrading col-lagen, these enzymes break down an important mechanical barrier that normally stands in the way of metastasis. We remain ignorant of the complex array of genes that directly or indi-rectly orchestrates this release of collagenase and other degradative enzymes and thereby advances the metastatic process.

But metastasis involves more than the breakdown of barriers that impede tumor ex-pansion. Early in the process, individual cells must disengage from the contacts that normally bind them to their neighbors. Later, these migrant cells must attach themselves to a new set of cells in a completely different tissue.

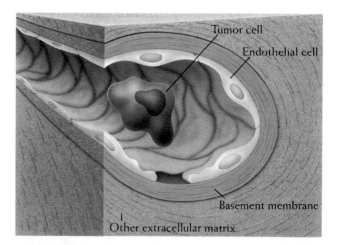

Tumor cell

Endothelial cell

Basement membrane

Other extracellular matrix

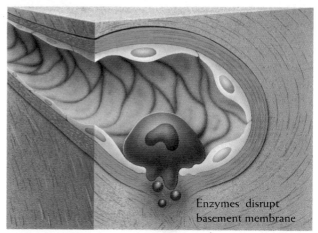

Enzymes disrupt basement membrane

Invasion is the complex process that allows tumor cells to escape from the circulation and establish metastases in tissues. As a prelude to invasion, a tumor cell in-duces the endothelial cells that line the blood vessels to retract, exposing the matrix of proteins called the base-ment membrane (top). After attaching to the basement membrane by binding certain molecules on it, enzymes secreted by the cell cleave the matrix proteins and cut a hole in the membrane (center). The tumor cell then moves into the hole while continuing to produce more enzymes that allow it to penetrate the layers of extra-cellular material beyond the basement membrane (bot-tom) and enter the tissues.

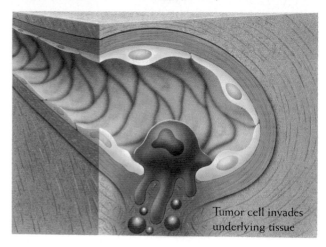

Tumor cell invades underlying tissue

Relationships in both the primary organ and the distant site depend upon direct physical contact between cells. We now know that a cell becomes tethered to its surroundings by a distinct set of cell surface receptors, which provide a mechanical link between the cell's cytoskeleton and molecules outside the cell, including components of the extracellular matrix as well as surface molecules on neighboring cells.

Some evidence on this point comes from a class of surface receptors known as cadherins, which form direct bridges between similar cells. When normal dog-kidney epithelial cells are prevented from displaying their cell surface E-cadherin molecules—for example, by inserting a viral oncogene into these cells—they become uncharacteristically migratory and even invasive. Forcing these virus-transformed cells to reexpress E-cadherin (by inserting extra E-cadherin genes into them) deprives them of their invasive properties.

Another class of cell surface receptors, the integrins, enables a cell to adhere tightly to extracellular matrix molecules. Certain rodent cells require $\alpha_5\beta_1$ integrin to bind to their normal extracellular matrix. When transformed into tumor cells, they display less $\alpha_5\beta_1$ on their surface and may make a novel integrin instead. Invasive melanomas, for example, display increased amounts of $\alpha_\nu\beta_3$ integrin, which apparently permits them to adhere to the types of extracellular matrix found in the organs that they colonize. Modulation of these cell surface receptors, which seems to play an important role in metastasis, may resemble events that occur early in embryogenesis to allow the programmed migration of cells to various parts of the developing organism.

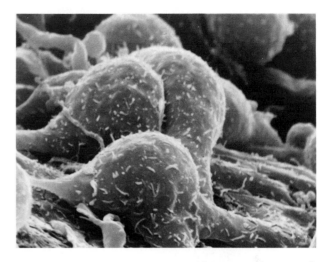

Metastatic melanoma cell.

The molecular and biochemical tools currently in hand are so powerful that each step in growth deregulation and metastasis should yield to the concerted efforts of researchers in the coming decade. It is likely that by the year 2000 we will have gained insight into most of the molecular and biochemical steps involved in the development of at least one human cancer. Soon thereafter, the complex life histories of a number of cancer types may become clear.

By then, we should know exactly how many genetic changes are required to make a malignant cancer cell and how each alteration of the cellular genome creates the biochemical shifts that confer growth advantage on the evolving tumor. When these molecular processes in the cancer cell are revealed, they will become targets for whole new generations of compounds synthesized to block or disrupt them, stopping the malignant growth. These hopeful clinical prospects fuel extra excitement in this rapidly moving field of science.

A regional cancer treatment center in Toulouse, France, publicizes its consultation hours (1932).

CANCER GENES
IN THE CLINIC

In the preceding chapters, we have recounted some of the extraordinary recent advances in understanding cancer at the cellular and molecular levels. But now we must confront a dismaying fact about cancer as a human disease: incidence and mortality have changed very little over the past few decades, despite our greatly expanded knowledge. Why have we failed to translate what we know into a better outlook for those who have experienced cancer or are destined to develop it? What are the prospects for improving the situation in the future?

It is very unlikely that we will ever be entirely free of the threat of death from cancer. The disease is common, afflicting at least one-quarter of the inhabitants of developed countries; it can affect virtually any of our cell lineages through mutations that cannot be completely avoided; and the targets of malignant mutations are indispensable genes whose normal products are essential for growth and development. Together, these features create pragmatic and theoretical obstacles—biological, medical, and ethical—to the goal of eliminating cancer from human society.

Even in our less than ideal world, however, we can envision great improvements in our current approaches to the control of cancer. In principle, control can be exerted at four levels: (1) identification of genetic predispositions to cancer, followed by intensive monitoring of those at risk; (2) reduction of exposure to environmental oncogenic agents, including viruses and chemical and physical carcinogens; (3) early and precise diagnosis of premalignant and malignant change; and (4) effective treatment by removal or destruction of cancer cells once they appear.

ASSESSING GENETIC RISK

Some individuals are at especially high risk for one or several kinds of cancer because of their genetic makeup. The chances of developing cancer can be reduced in some of these cases by routine monitoring for incipient tumors with the use of sensitive diagnostic procedures at frequent intervals (for example, examination for retinoblastoma in children known to harbor mutant Rb genes) or by avoidance of certain mutagens (for example, sunlight in xeroderma pigmentosum patients). Until recently, however, it was difficult to make initial identifica-

tion of individuals at risk unless they were members of a family known to transmit genes predisposing to a particular type of cancer. Even then, it was often not possible to know whether a given member of such a family was genetically predisposed, since the responsible mutant gene had not been identified and isolated by molecular cloning.

Even with the currently available genetic techniques, substantial problems still remain, as is made apparent by studying retinoblastoma (Chapter 5). We can now, in principle, test for a mutant gene in an individual's DNA because the Rb gene has been cloned and its normal sequence determined. Such screening is of great practical value because frequent examination of patients identified to be at risk and laser removal of any small tumors can prevent loss of vision, disfigurement, and invasive disease. Since retinoblastomas are uncommon after the age of four, successful surveillance and treatment in early life have especially great rewards.

Yet retinoblastoma is rare, and only one-third of patients have an inherited form of the disease, so it is not practical to test the entire population for genetic susceptibility; screening is confined to children with siblings, parents, or other close relatives who have had multiple retinoblastomas. New germline mutations occur fairly often in the Rb gene, however, and a substantial number of newborns who inherit a mutant gene will lack a family history of the disease and so will not be considered for genetic testing. Thus only about 10 percent of cases—20 to 30 per year in the United States—are likely to be predicted by molecular tests.

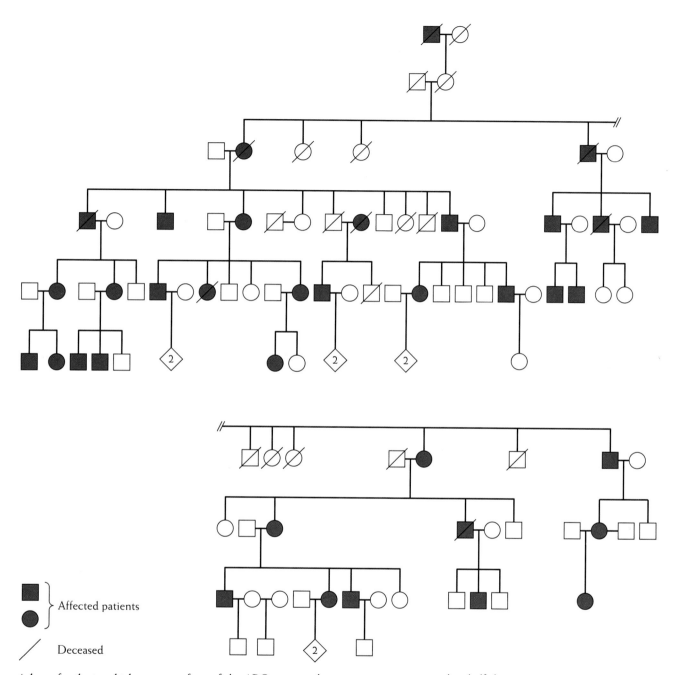

■ } Affected patients
●

╱ Deceased

A large family in which a mutant form of the APC gene on chromosome 5q is transmitted to half the offspring of individuals who have polyposis of the colon. Since the APC gene has been cloned, a diagnosis can be made with molecular tests early in life, before colon polyps or cancers appear.

Even in families selected for known risk, the tests are problematic and expensive. The Rb gene is very large—180,000 base pairs long—and any one of a large number of distinct mutations may be encountered in affected families. Thus an elaborate study of the Rb genes from one or both parents may be needed to design a suitable test.

Similar considerations apply to other situations in which an inherited mutation of a specific cancer gene is known to predispose strongly to certain tumors. Detailed analysis of three recently isolated tumor suppressor genes—the familial adenomatous polyposis coli (APC) gene on chromosome 5, the neurofibromatosis-1 (NF-1) gene on chromosome 17, and the Wilms' tumor-1 (WT-1) gene on chromosome 11—can often identify individuals at risk of developing the associated tumors in families with established disease histories. But these genes have been available for molecular scrutiny too short a time to evaluate their clinical utility fully.

Considerable efforts are being made to identify additional genes that, in mutant form, confer susceptibility to common cancers. For example, the appearance of breast cancer before menopause strongly correlates in many families with the inheritance of alleles of a still-unidentified gene on the long arm of chromosome 17. Overall, about 5 percent of breast cancers are linked to this gene. Susceptibilities to several rarer diseases associated with benign or malignant tumors (multiple endocrine adenomatosis, Beckwith-Wiedemann syndrome, and others) also have been ascribed to genetic transmission of chromosomal segments presumed to harbor mutant tumor suppressor genes. Once isolated, study of such genes may show them to be inherited in mutant form more often than is currently suspected. Thus, these genes might be found to be responsible for a far larger number of tumors than thought at present.

In the future, far-reaching genetic assessments of an individual's cancer risk might be based upon a profile of several cancer-related loci. Such a composite analysis could perhaps project one's likelihood of developing any of the common human cancers at different stages of life. There may also be single genes that in mutant form predispose to a variety of cancers. Most intriguing in this regard is the remarkable discovery that mutant p53 genes are inherited in families with the so-called Li-Fraumeni syndrome. Affected members have an especially high incidence of several relatively common cancers, such as breast carcinomas, connective tissue sarcomas, and brain tumors, and disease may occur at any time from childhood to old age.

Although identified Li-Fraumeni families are rare, many other families may inherit mutations—in p53 or other genes—that place them at a significantly higher than average risk for one or more forms of cancer. It is often difficult to identify those families with hereditary factors that cause an increased susceptibility to cancer: cancer is common and families often have multiple cases just by random chance. Upon occasion, screening families for mutant forms of already well-studied genes uncovers useful markers for disease risk. Once again, the p53 gene proves illustrative. Recent studies show that some patients may be predisposed to sarcomas, even without a family his-

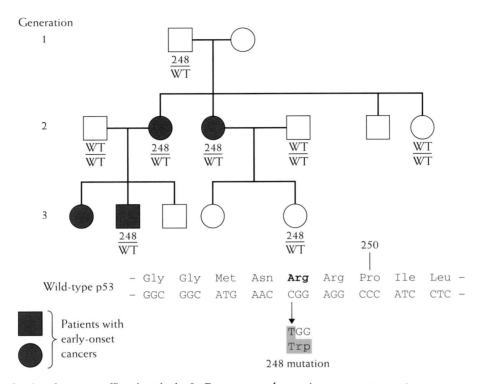

A pedigree for a family of patients afflicted with the Li-Fraumeni syndrome. A mutant p53 gene is associated with a predisposition to early-onset cancers.

tory of the Li-Fraumeni syndrome, because they have inherited a mutant copy of the p53 gene. Probably no more than 1 to 2 percent of all patients with sarcomas carry an inherited mutant p53 gene, but by identifying such individuals it would be possible for researchers to monitor them, as well as their relatives who carry the same allele, for the development of cancer.

Another type of definable genetic predisposition to cancer is represented by several diseases in which somatic mutations occur at abnormally high rates. This condition has been documented most graphically in families with xeroderma pigmentosum (XP). Affected individuals inherit two mutant copies of one of the several genes required to repair DNA damage caused by exposure to the UV radiation in sunlight. As a consequence, UV-induced DNA damage goes unrepaired, and mutations accumulate in the skin cells. The skin cancers that then appear at high rates often carry mutations in p53 genes that are typical of UV-induced damage. Because two of the several defective DNA repair genes have now been isolated from patients with different forms of XP, newborns in affected families can, in theory, be tested for inheritance of mutant alleles.

Despite these advances, the prospects for assessment of cancer risk pose difficult problems. How much should we be willing to spend to predict a twofold, tenfold, or hundredfold increase in cancer risk? Should everyone be tested, or only those with a suspicious family history? Can the tests be designed to identify a large proportion of those who will develop cancer, not just the very small segment of the population—currently much less than 1 percent—at risk for the rare malignant syndromes discussed here? If such genetic tests are found to be accurate predictors of risk, will the information they yield be acted upon in useful ways—for example, with sensitive tests to screen for tumors at very early stages and to treat them with effective therapies once they are detected? Or will individuals deemed to be at even moderate risk be stigmatized when seeking employment, insurance, or a mate? Can the information gathered by testing be kept confidential? In short, will generating a large amount of predictive information increase our well-being and life expectancy? Or will our society become cancer-obsessed rather than cancer-free?

REDUCING ENVIRONMENTAL MUTAGENS

Studies summarized in Chapter 3 have helped to identify components of our environment that foster mutations, some of which affect cancer genes and thereby promote neoplastic disease. The factors implicated include many items in our diet, particularly high-fat meats;

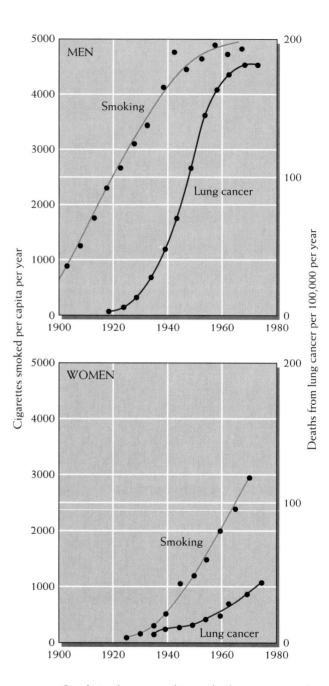

Correlation between smoking and subsequent rise in the death rate from lung cancer, for men and women in England.

agents such as tobacco and alcohol, industrial pollutants, and X-ray or UV radiation; and certain viruses. Do such lists offer grounds for optimism or pessimism? On the one hand, individuals should be able to avoid contact with many of the agents associated with a high risk of cancer, and vaccines may be produced that protect human beings against infection by oncogenic viruses. On the other hand, the oncogenic effects of food and drink seem nearly impossible to avoid, and long-standing warnings against some of the most potent carcinogenic agents have only moderately curtailed their use.

The history of tobacco use provides a sobering view of society's limited capacity to capitalize upon scientific progress and improve human health through preventive measures. Although epidemiological studies in the 1940s and 1950s established a close association between smoking and various carcinomas, and although this evidence was promulgated by the U.S. Surgeon-General as early as 1964, the incidence of smoking has declined significantly only in the past few years and only in certain parts of the population. In fact, the use of tobacco products continues to rise among women and certain ethnic and socioeconomic groups. As a result, carcinoma of the lung, an especially difficult cancer to treat, has recently surpassed carcinoma of the breast as the most common cancer in American women.

This saga should remind us that important discoveries about the molecular origins and

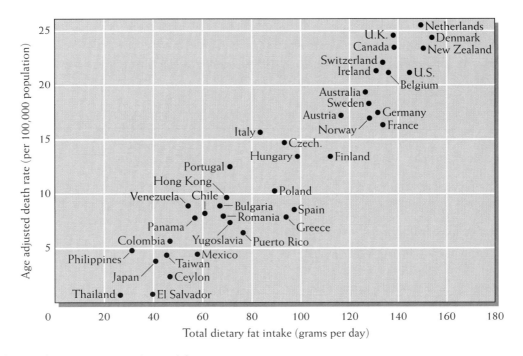

Correlation between breast cancer mortality and fat consumption in various countries.

environmental causes of cancer do not automatically provide health benefits, even when apparently simple countermeasures are required. Attempts are being made to restrict exposure to various environmental carcinogens. Individuals, particularly fair-skinned ones, are being urged to avoid sunlight and thereby decrease the incidence of skin cancers known to be associated with UV-induced mutations. Similar efforts are being made to influence dietary patterns—for example, by restricting the intake of fat to lower the incidence of carcinomas of the colon and rectum. These efforts are difficult to sustain, however, because of conflicting claims about the strength of the evidence and because pleasurable habits are not easily given up.

Epidemiological control is generally most effective when laws limit the use of carcinogenic materials by industry. Prohibition of radium in watch dials and asbestos in manufacturing and shipyards is generally considered to have been successful in decreasing bladder cancer and mesotheliomas, respectively, in exposed workers. Such legislation is often difficult to enact, however, because the data are incomplete or conflicting or because powerful financial interests are threatened.

Viruses linked to human cancers are attractive targets of efforts to prevent tumors through immunization against viral infection. For example, although the genetic mechanisms by which hepatitis B virus induces liver cancer remain incompletely understood, the association between the two is strong enough to argue that prevention of HBV infection should dramatically reduce the frequency of this tumor, currently the most common lethal cancer in Southeast Asia and parts of Africa. Because HBV infection in these areas usually occurs during delivery, by transmission from the blood of infected mothers, an effective vaccine must be active soon after birth. Yet the success of this anticancer strategy can be assessed only by following a large cohort of vaccinated patients for as long as 50 years, since hepatocellular carcinoma generally appears between the ages of 40 and 60. This strategy became possible about 10 years ago, with the production of HBV vaccines through recombinant DNA technology. During the past decade, large-scale field trials have been initiated in Southeast Asia and Africa, with early results indicating that these vaccines prevent chronic HBV infection in over 90 percent of the offspring of infected women. It will, of course, take many more years to determine whether those vaccinated show the hoped-for decrease in liver cancer.

The outlook for a similar strategy to prevent the other three virus-associated human

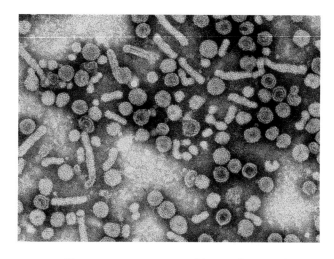

Electron microscope view of human hepatitis B virus.

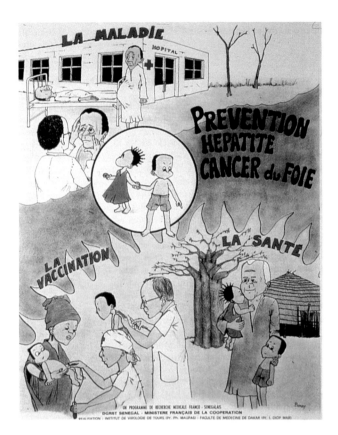

A poster from a campaign to vaccinate newborn infants against hepatitis B virus—and thereby prevent liver cancer much later.

virus. For all of these viruses, as for HBV, it will require many years to gauge the effectiveness of any vaccine. Moreover, possible benefits must be weighed against the safety of any vaccine ultimately developed. At present, the emphasis is on identifying individuals chronically infected with oncogenic viruses, so that they can be carefully monitored for the first signs of cancer and so that transmission of

cancers is less promising. As yet, there are no effective vaccines against human herpesviruses (EBV), papilloma viruses (HPV 16 and 18), or retroviruses (HTLV-1). Mounting large-scale vaccination efforts may be deterred by the fact that the likelihood of any infected individual developing cancer is low. In parts of Japan, for instance, 20 percent or more of the population may be chronically infected with HTLV-1, but less than 5 percent of those infected will ever develop the T-cell leukemia associated with the

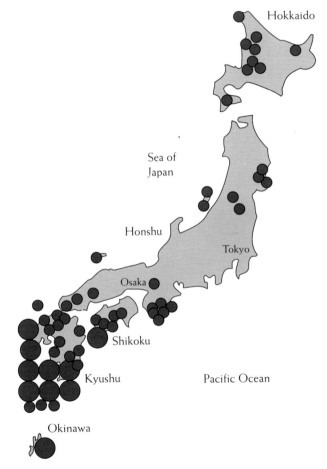

Map of Japan showing distribution of T-cell leukemia. The larger the dots, the more cases.

HTLV-1, HBV, and EBV by blood transfusion can be avoided.

The intense efforts currently under way to produce an effective drug and a vaccine against human immunodeficiency virus (HIV) could also affect the incidence of certain cancers commonly encountered in patients with AIDS—particularly Kaposi's sarcoma and B-cell lymphoma. HIV does not trigger these cancers directly: it does not carry a viral oncogene, and viral DNA cannot be found in the tumor cells. Instead, these cancers may arise because of compromises to the immune system or because of growth factors produced by noncancerous cells infected by the virus. Regardless of the oncogenic mechanism, a reduction of AIDS-associated cancers would be a welcome secondary effect of successful control of HIV.

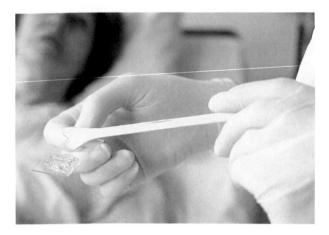

Above: A physician takes a Pap smear of cells from the uterine cervix. At right: Microscopic view of cells taken from an asymptomatic patient suggests the diagnosis of an early and treatable stage of cervical carcinoma.

IMPROVING DIAGNOSIS

Early diagnosis of a cancer or a precancerous condition offers many advantages. In early stages, only a small number of cells is involved, and the abnormal cells are unlikely to have invaded local tissues or metastasized. It is usually possible, at this stage, to cure a patient by simple surgical removal of the unwanted cells or by local irradiation to kill them. These benefits are most often achieved when tumors are suspected and can be sought regularly (such as in familial retinoblastoma); when premalignant growths can be found with relatively simple procedures (such as Pap smears to look for abnormal cells shed from the uterine cervix); and when tumors are readily visible (such as skin cancers). Early diagnosis of many of the most common and aggressive cancers remains frustrated, however, because methods for early detection either do not exist (for example, tumors of the brain and pancreas) or are inconvenient or imperfect (for example, carcinomas of the breast and colon). By the time such

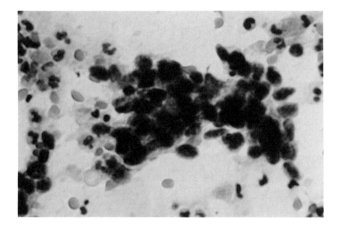

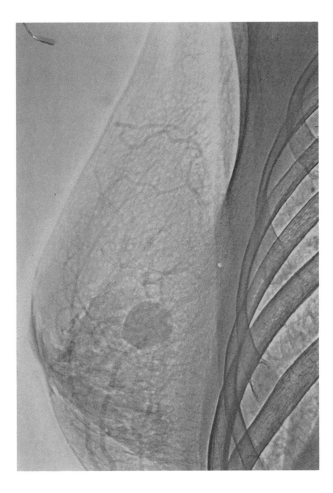

tumors produce clinical symptoms, they have already grown to form masses of 10^{10} (ten thousand million) cells or more; even when they can be detected with current screening procedures such as mammography and colonoscopy, they are nearly as large, although often still curable.

Can new knowledge about the molecular basis of cancer facilitate earlier diagnosis? Techniques such as the polymerase chain reaction (PCR) can detect a mutation in the DNA obtained from a single cell; several common mutations of proto-oncogenes and tumor suppressor genes have been identified in human cancers; and certain of these mutations have been regularly associated with certain cancers. Nevertheless, such conceptual and technical advances offer few advantages in current medical practice. It is simply impractical to sample most internal organs for mutant cells, and it would be prohibitively expensive to screen the whole population regularly for even the most common mutations, should suitable samples become easily obtainable. One response to this problem might exploit the fact that some of the major sites for cancer—the lungs, intestines, kidneys, and bladder—are continually shedding cells into excreted materials—sputum, feces, and urine—that are, in principle, available for highly sensitive tests. Recent trials using the PCR method to detect mutant ras genes in cells present in feces have identified patients who proved to have sizable adenomas or carcinomas of the large intestine. It is, however, premature to say whether PCR tests will ever become routine screening devices for cancer of the intestine, lungs, or urinary tract.

Molecular techniques also promise more precise and informative diagnoses, and such methods are already in use in a few clinical situations. For instance, the classification of leukemia—and consequently the choice of treat-

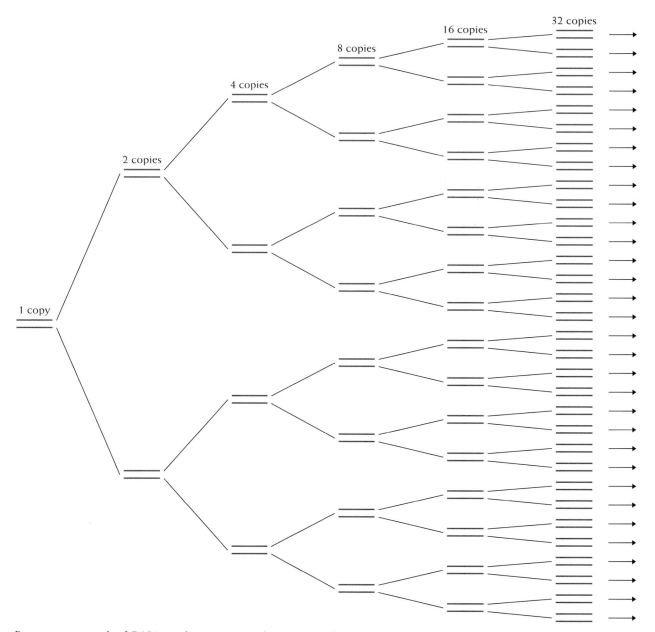

By successive rounds of DNA synthesis in a test tube, even a single DNA molecule can be amplified sufficiently (e.g., 100-million-fold) to be detected and analyzed by conventional procedures. This so-called polymerase chain reaction (PCR) is based upon the use of specific "primers" that restrict DNA synthesis to sequences adjacent to those recognized by the primers. The PCR method now has numerous applications in medicine, biotechnology, and basic research.

ment—may be strongly influenced by the kind of chromosomal translocation found in the tumors. The Philadelphia chromosome, emblematic of certain myeloid and lymphoid leukemias (Chapters 3 and 4), is more easily detected by molecular tests for an abnormal abl proto-oncogene than by traditional microscopic inspection of chromosomes. Moreover, the sensitivity of these tests now permits physicians to monitor patients who have undergone rigorous therapy—including bone marrow transplantation—for persistence or regrowth of even very small numbers of leukemic cells.

Tests for mutant oncogenes and tumor suppressor genes can also help evaluate abnormalities that may be precancerous. For instance, some patients with a chronic abnormality of blood-cell differentiation called myelodysplastic syndrome eventually develop a life-threatening leukemia. The minority of patients most likely to experience leukemia can be identified by observing whether or not mutations have occurred at certain positions within the ras genes in the premalignant cells. Women with abnormal Pap smears are often infected with human papilloma viruses, but only a few types of HPV confer high risk of cervical carcinomas; products of the type 16 and 18 viruses interfere potently with the products of two of the infected cell's tumor suppressor genes (Rb and p53). Thus, virus typing with molecular tools may give information about the risk of cancer and suggest therapy for a condition that is not yet unambiguously malignant.

Even when a full-fledged cancer has been diagnosed by conventional means, newly developed molecular tests can predict its severity, categorize it more precisely, and guide the choice of therapy. Leukemic cells from patients with acute promyelocytic leukemia often have a translocation chromosome formed from the joining of a part of chromosome 15 to a part

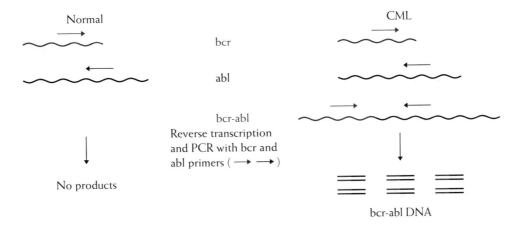

Detection of bcr-abl hybrid messenger RNA using the polymer chain reaction technique. The PCR method is a sensitive test for the Philadelphia chromosome.

of chromosome 17. This results in the generation of a novel transcription factor containing part of the protein derived from the normal receptor for retinoic acid, which is related to vitamin A. Remarkably, patients with this particular translocation experience a rapid and often long-lived remission when treated with retinoic acid. Thus, specific testing for the translocation once leukemia has been diagnosed can have important clinical consequences.

The N-myc proto-oncogene is frequently amplified during the genesis of neuroblastoma, one of the most common cancers of young children (Chapter 4). An increase in the number of N-myc gene copies can be measured quite easily by using specific radioactive DNA probes and observing the intensity of bands produced on an X-ray film. About one-third of surveyed neuroblastomas are found to have amplified N-myc genes, and such amplification is highly predictive of an unfavorable prognosis. Most patients with this amplification are already at an advanced stage of disease that is likely to be lethal regardless of whether N-myc is amplified; at this stage, measurement of gene copy number provides no special insight into prognosis. Patients with apparently less advanced disease are usually cured by chemotherapy; in them, discovery of an amplified N-myc gene is ominous, portending aggressive disease and a poor response to conventional therapy.

Unfortunately, the more refined cancer diagnoses now possible through tests for mutant genes have not yet provided clinically useful information in most situations (neuroblastomas and a few leukemias are exceptions). Even for tumors in which certain oncogenic mutations are frequently encountered (see Chapter 7 for examples), informative correlations have not yet emerged—which is especially disappointing given the precision and elegance of these diagnostic tests.

For these reasons, the detection of mutant cancer genes is not yet a common component of clinical oncology. Current diagnostic methods are based largely upon the pathologist's

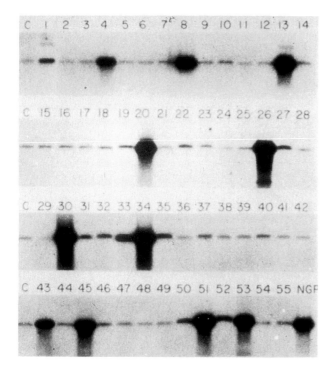

A survey of neuroblastoma DNA from several patients for amplification of the N-myc gene. The common relatively thin band indicates the normal two copies of the gene; the dark bands show various degrees of amplification, up to hundreds of copies per cell.

survey of tumor samples, using microscopic criteria that have changed little over several decades. It seems inevitable that the more precise methods made possible by descriptions of the molecular basis of cancer will ultimately affect diagnosis profoundly. But it may be years before the tests are simple enough and the interpretations certain enough to replace time-honored methods. Only long-term observation of patients with tumors that carry specific sets of mutated genes will provide the answers to the most pressing questions: Are certain mutations, or combinations of mutations, associated with a favorable clinical outcome or a favorable response to certain therapies? Do recurrent combinations of mutations occur in preferred orders, and do they predict the likelihood of a future disease course such as metastasis?

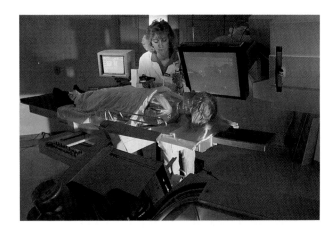

A patient undergoes radiotherapy for cancer.

TREATING CANCER

Current strategies for cancer therapy are based upon a large body of empirical observations in the clinic that lacks any connection to the genetic abnormalities that produce the cancers. The strategies do not address the underlying causes of disease but instead use methods that have worked in the past to remove or kill as many cancer cells as possible while minimizing damage to normal tissue. This approach achieves its greatest success when surgery can be employed to eradicate a tumor that has not metastasized from a primary site—particularly a site that can be sacrificed without major disability, such as a segment of skin, colon, or breast. Substantial rates of cure, with only modest degrees of disfigurement, are also possible with localized tumors in more critical organs, especially when the tumors are known to be particularly sensitive to the cell-killing effects of radiation. Chemotherapy is often used in combination with surgery or radiation to eliminate surviving cancer cells, especially potential metastases.

Even when widespread and unsuitable for local surgery or radiation, some tumors—particularly certain leukemias, lymphomas, and sarcomas—may respond extremely well to chemotherapy. The drugs currently in use are chosen, often in combination, because clinical experience has shown each drug or combination to be the most effective in killing certain types of cancer cells. Most of these drugs are so-called metabolic inhibitors: they interfere with the ability of any growing cell to make more DNA or to divide its chromosomes into daughter cells. Methotrexate, for example, inhibits the enzyme dihydrofolate reductase, required in all cells for production of the deoxynucleotides used to synthesize DNA. Other agents, such as vincristine, bind to the cytoskeletal components of the mitotic spindle and thereby prevent chromosomal separation during cell division. Yet other types of drugs, such as adriamycin, wedge themselves between the nucleotide bases in DNA or attack the bases chemically; as a result, they may either break the chains or modify the information content. Many of these drugs enter the body in an inactive form and must be acted upon by some of the same systems required to activate the chemical carcinogens, as described in Chapter 3; this is perhaps not surprising, since carcinogens and chemotherapeutic agents often have common properties and mechanisms. Indeed, many drugs used in chemotherapy are mutagenic and inherently carcinogenic.

Whatever their mode of action, the drugs used for chemotherapy do not attack cancer cells with great precision; they are also toxic for normal tissues, particularly the bone marrow, the hair follicles, and the mucosal surfaces of the mouth, throat, and intestine—the places where tissue integrity depends upon constant cell growth and division. This is why chemotherapy is routinely accompanied by hair loss, sores, diarrhea, and depletion of the normal cellular components of the blood; indeed, it is usual to administer antineoplastic drugs until some or all of these signs of toxicity appear, in order to achieve the greatest possible reduction in the number of cancer cells. (In a few cancers—including cancers of the breast, ovary, and prostate—less toxic drugs, such as hormonal agents, are at least partially effective.)

The most important of these toxic side effects affect the bone marrow. The loss of red-blood-cell precursors causes anemia and poor oxygen-carrying capacity, the loss of white cells impairs immune response, and the loss of platelets affects blood clotting. Patients undergoing chemotherapy are at special risk of bleeding; life-threatening infection by viruses, bacteria, and fungi; and (particularly in older patients) strokes and heart failure. Some of these risks can be reduced significantly by frequent transfusion of whole blood or components of blood (platelets or red or white cells). Damaged bone marrow can now be replaced by reinfusion of the patient's own marrow, prepared and stored away before therapy, or marrow from a compatible donor; this allows extremely high and potentially curative doses of cytotoxic drugs to be used. The recent commercial production of hematopoietic growth and differentiation factors using recombinant DNA technology has improved the chances of recovery after chemotherapy, with or without bone marrow transplantation. By promoting the survival, proliferation, and maturation of blood-cell precursors that have survived chemotherapy, these factors hasten regeneration of essential cell types in the blood.

Even if patients can be protected against the toxic effects of chemotherapy, the regimen may fail because the cancer cells are insufficiently sensitive to the drugs employed. Resistance to chemotherapy often appears during the course of treatment because cancer cells de-

Another Side of Drug Resistance

An especially invidious form of resistance to chemotherapy occurs when cancer cells amplify a gene called MDR (for multiple drug resistance). The large protein made by the MDR gene works as a chemical pump at the plasma membrane to rid the cell of several kinds of chemicals, including several of the most effective cancer drugs.

As discussed earlier, cancer cells seem prone to replicate portions of their DNA multiple times within a single cell cycle, leading to gene amplification. Indeed, amplification of certain proto-oncogenes can confer substantial growth advantage on a cell. Analogously, if a cancer cell in a patient being treated with an effective chemotherapeutic drug amplifies its MDR gene, it will acquire a competitive growth advantage, since it can more efficiently pump out the toxic drug—and many other potentially useful therapeutic agents as well.

On the other hand, it may soon be possible to take advantage of MDR protein overproduction to aid in cancer chemotherapy, using this protein to protect normal bone marrow cells from the toxic effects of chemotherapy and thereby increase the amount of drug a patient could tolerate. This could be achieved by delivering extra copies of the MDR gene to hematopoietic cells in retroviral vectors (see page 204) before the initiation of chemotherapy. The protected cells would serve to replenish blood cells after therapy.

velop additional mutations that make them impervious to drug molecules. These mutations may change the amino acid sequence of enzymes the drugs are intended to inhibit, or amplify a gene whose protein product, in excessive amounts, pumps the drugs out of the tumor cell. Regardless of the mechanism, the resistant cell has achieved a growth advantage over its siblings in the presence of the anti-cancer drugs. Ultimately, such cells and their progeny will proliferate and become, by natural selection, the predominant components of the cancer.

Despite its sometimes spectacular successes with certain cancers, the overall verdict on chemotherapy is not favorable, and the five-year survival rates for most tumors have not improved significantly in the years since drugs were first widely used. It is natural, then, to inquire whether new, more specific therapies can be devised by taking advantage of what is now known about genetic abnormalities of the cancer cell, particularly those that lead to local invasion and to metastatic colonization.

There are at least three ways to exploit our new understanding of cancer cells. The first is to use distinctive properties of tumor cells to ensure that cytotoxic agents are delivered preferentially to the cancerous target cells rather than to normal cells. This may well be achieved most readily by taking advantage of the appearance of novel or unusually abundant proteins on the cancer cell surface. For example, amplification of genes encoding cell surface receptors, mutations that change the character of a cell surface protein, or alterations in the control of a receptor gene could produce a cancer cell easily distinguished from virtually all others. Lethal molecules such as bacterial toxins, linked to antibodies or ligands that bind to specific cell surface proteins, could then be concentrated on cancer cells, damaging or killing them but affecting other cells minimally. Such strategies have been effective against some cancers in animals and are being developed for clinical trials in human beings.

A second approach is to interfere with a signaling pathway that displays exaggerated activity in a cancer cell. Thus we might hope to slow the growth of cancer cells by, for example, blocking an overproduced autocrine growth factor, inhibiting an overactive protein-tyrosine kinase, switching off a mutant ras protein that is frozen in the active state, or reversing the effects of an overactive transcription factor. Unfortunately, drugs are not yet available to do most of these things, even in cell extracts or culture, let alone in living organisms. Development of such drugs will be especially challenging because they need to penetrate tumor cells; this requirement limits the range of chemicals that are suitable, since the plasma membrane that surrounds all animal cells is designed to limit the entrance of most compounds. Entry is generally restricted to

small molecules having a minimum of electric charge (absence of charge allows them to slip through the fatty membrane) or to those that can penetrate the cell using existing, specialized import mechanisms. The introduction into cells of much larger molecules—specific antibodies, other proteins, or polynucleotides—to counteract the effects of oncogenic mutations will require novel delivery systems.

There is an additional important concern about attempts to interfere with cell signaling: the pathways to be inhibited are also crucial to the well-being of normal cells, so any drugs effective against tumors are likely to be just as toxic for normal cells as those currently used in chemotherapy. It might be possible, however, to identify drugs that block the activity of mutant signaling proteins but not their normal versions. Also, pharmacology is rich with examples of drugs that inhibit normal processes—including hormonal signaling and activities of the central nervous system—yet can be administered to patients in a way that produces major benefits with few side effects.

The third possible therapy is to replace the functions normally supplied by a tumor suppressor gene that has been inactivated during malignant development. In principle, the simplest strategy is to substitute for the inactive tumor suppressor gene by infecting the cancer cells with a virus (see page 204) carrying a normal copy of the gene; normal cells, already carrying two copies of such a gene, would presumably tolerate additional copies introduced by the viral vector. The cancer cells, in contrast, should respond by returning to a more normal pattern of growth. In practice there are some obvious, but perhaps not insurmountable, problems. Since it will be impossible to deliver the missing gene to all the tumor cells, and difficult to deliver it to even the majority, only a modest and transient decline in the number of actively growing cancer cells is likely to be achieved. In combination with other kinds of therapy, however, delivery to even 80 percent of tumor cells might have a significant effect on the clinical outcome. Recent studies of cancer cell lines in culture provide grounds for optimism: it appears that replacing a missing tumor suppressor gene can sometimes reverse the cancer-forming potential even of cells with multiple genetic lesions. This suggests that the cancer phenotype may depend simultaneously on the effects of each of these mutations, and the cell may revert to normal if any one of them is corrected.

These three general approaches, emerging directly from the genetic alterations described in this book, all warrant further attention, regardless of their inherent problems. Alternative strategies based upon new insights into the mechanisms governing the cell division cycle, DNA damage, and immune responses to tumors also show promise and need study. For example, the cytotoxic effects of the metabolic inhibitors in current use depend heavily upon perturbations of the cell cycle; when DNA synthesis is inhibited in cycling cells, cell death is most likely to occur if the cells proceed through mitosis without completely duplicating their chromosomes. As described in Chapter 1, normal cells exercise controls that prevent division before DNA replication is complete. If cancer cells can be induced to

relax such controls, they will be more severely affected by the metabolic inhibitors and thus more vulnerable to chemotherapy.

Another avenue to more potent intervention might be possible through a greater understanding of the processes that cause mutation in cancer cells. We have seen that cancer is a multistep process in which as many as five to ten mutations may be required to achieve maximal oncogenic capacity. The probabilities that any single cell will accumulate such a large number of mutations are vanishingly small, unless the cell has undergone some fundamental change that increases the mutation frequency (see Chapter 7). If such changes can be comprehended in detail, it may be possible to accelerate the mutation rate still further, increasing it to a point at which the accumulated mutations cripple the cancer cell, rather than merely stripping it of restraints on its growth.

Finally, there is renewed interest in the topic of immune response to cancers. Arguments about whether the immune system functions as a surveillance device that defends an organism against the development of many cancers over a lifetime have raged for years without satisfactory resolution. There is clear evidence, however, that immune cells are commonly present in tumors and that they are often directed against antigens displayed on the tumor cells. Some of these immune cells can damage or even kill the antigen-displaying tumor cells and one day may be mobilized as highly effective weapons to wipe out large numbers of cancer cells in the body of the patient.

Retroviral Vectors in Gene Therapy

H ow might we replace missing genes or install new, beneficial ones? The development in the 1970s of methods for the molecular cloning of genes inspired thinking about what has come to be called gene therapy.

What is the best way to deliver genes to human cells? As we have seen in previous chapters, retroviruses often carry oncogenes derived from normal cellular genes; they are naturally occurring genetic vectors. Because they have many features desirable in a gene transporter—efficient integration into host chromosomes, relative simplicity of design, and no toxic effects

upon infected cells—retroviruses have been vigorously manipulated to produce excellent vectors, some of which are already being used in clinical trials in patients with cancer or metabolic disorders. (To avoid disturbing the human germ line, and hence subsequent generations, in unanticipated ways, acceptable strategies must be designed exclusively for somatic cells.)

The strategies employed for retroviral vectoring depend upon a single important fact: the viral proteins in an infectious particle can be provided by genes that are not actually present in the particle. Two components are required to create viral vector

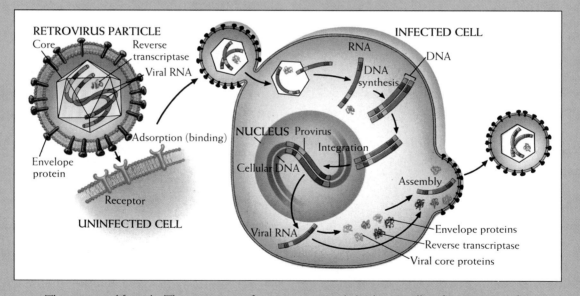

The retrovirus life cycle. The protein coat of a retrovirus particle binds to a cell surface receptor. After uncoating within the cytoplasm, the viral core is the site of reverse transcription. (The drawing omits the core to display the conversion of retroviral RNA to DNA.) This DNA provirus, integrated into the cell chromosome, directs synthesis of progeny retrovirus components.

particles that can infect and express their genes in desired target cells: (1) a so-called helper cell, equipped with genes that produce the viral proteins from which the vector virus particle is assembled, and (2) a recombinant retroviral genome, which includes the desired (cellular) genes and the viral signals that ensure assembly into the vector. Because the vector genome does not carry its own viral genes, the infected target cell will make only the protein encoded by the delivered nonviral gene and cannot proceed to make further virus particles. As a consequence, the vector can be directed at critical target cells and will not spread from them to other, potentially irrelevant cells.

Gene therapy is most obviously applicable to patients with inherited genetic deficiencies. But as this chapter has suggested, other goals for gene therapy are also possible: to protect normal bone marrow cells against drug toxicity; to replace missing tumor suppressor genes in cancer cells; and to stimulate immune cells to attack a tumor.

Retroviral vectors are assembled in cells designed to release only safe vectors. The helper cells synthesize viral proteins from RNA that cannot be packaged in virus particles. These proteins instead package vector RNA carrying therapeutic genes in the place of viral genes. The resulting particles can enter other cells, splice the therapeutic gene into cellular DNA, and produce therapeutic protein, but they cannot reproduce.

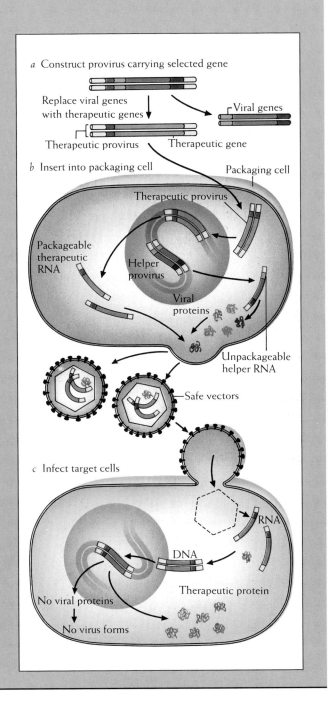

a Construct provirus carrying selected gene

Replace viral genes with therapeutic genes

Viral genes

Therapeutic provirus   Therapeutic gene

b Insert into packaging cell

Packaging cell

Therapeutic provirus

Packageable therapeutic RNA

Helper provirus

Viral proteins

Unpackageable helper RNA

Safe vectors

c Infect target cells

RNA

DNA

Therapeutic protein

No viral proteins

No virus forms

Innovative Therapies

Because cancer is so often a progressively lethal disease, it invites novel and even potentially dangerous therapies—some of which have performed with surprising success against particular forms of the disease, leading to significant improvements in care.

The work of William Coley illustrates some of the possibilities and problems. Exactly a hundred years ago Coley, a New York surgeon, initiated attempts to "vaccinate" cancer patients with mixtures of killed bacteria; his experiment was inspired by much earlier observations that some specific cancers appeared to enter remission if a patient contracted certain bacterial infections, particularly erysipelas (a streptococcal skin inflammation). Over the next 30 years "Coley's toxins," as they came to be called, induced remarkably long remissions in a substantial percentage of patients with soft-tissue sarcomas and lymphomas, although the treatment was far less successful with more common cancers like carcinomas. With the advent of radiation and chemotherapy, bacterial vaccines and their successes were largely forgotten.

Recent results have rekindled interest in the original findings and provided justification for pursuing newer, related therapies. The effectiveness of Coley's vaccines (or of the bacterial infections) is now thought to have been due to the production and release by normal cells of potent lymphocyte-specific growth and differentiation factors called cytokines. The cytokines—including tumor necrosis factors and several immune lymphokines—are thought to stimulate the proliferation and tumor-cell-killing activities of T lymphocytes and natural killer (NK) cells. Based upon these ideas, a number of clinical trials are currently under way; retroviral vectors, for example, are being used to insert cytokine genes into lymphocytes from cancer patients in the hope of activating immune reactivity against tumor cells.

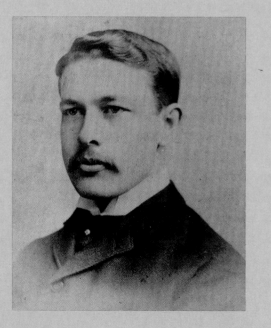

William Coley.

Can Cancer Be Eradicated?

For those of us privileged to study cancer, elimination of the disease is the ultimate goal. Yet a realistic view of the causes of cancer and their links to fundamental aspects of life—the mutagens in our environment and the genes required for normal growth and development— suggests that cancer is intrinsic to multicellular life and that the total eradication of cancer from our species is implausible.

Still, research on the origins of cancer must proceed with a mixture of optimism and reserve. On the one hand, we operate with the hope that to understand the disease will finally provide the means to control it. But we have also learned that even profound discoveries about the cause of disease do not invariably or immediately generate solutions. Louis Pasteur and Robert Koch, for example, established the bacterial origins of many common illnesses; but it was only decades later that their work was crowned by the discoveries of penicillin, streptomycin, and other antibiotics capable of subduing bacterial infections.

In the waning years of the twentieth century, it is excitement enough to begin to grasp the dimensions of cancerous change: the multitude of genes involved, the various ways in which their products affect growth, and the several pathways that lead to cancers in different tissues. New ideas about prevention, risk assessment, detection, diagnosis, and therapy are beginning to emerge, as this concluding chapter has indicated, based upon these glimmerings of comprehension.

As we emphasized at the outset of this volume, studying cancer at the level of cells and molecules has had effects that extend far beyond our understanding of this disease and its treatment in the clinic. The mechanisms that go awry in the development of a cancer cell are central to many biological processes, and insights gained into the lives of cancer cells deepen our understanding of many different aspects of human biology: our normal development, evolutionary origins, immune defenses, even aging and death. Cells, healthy and malignant, and the genes that control them, hold a key to what we are, where we came from, and what we one day may be.

SOURCES OF ILLUSTRATIONS

All line illustrations are by Fine Line Illustrations, Inc., and Network Graphics. Illustrations on pages 28, 150, 181, 182, 204, and 205 are by Tomo Narashima.

Frontispiece: National Library of Medicine.

Chapter 1 *Facing p. 1:* (top) David Scharf/Peter Arnold Inc.; (center left) Gerard Lacz/NHPA; (center right) Sample courtesy of William Sheridan, University of North Dakota, Grand Forks. Photo by Travis Amos. (bottom) M. A. L. Smith, Dept. of Horticulture, University of Illinois, Urbana. *p. 2, p. 3:* (top) Lennart Nilsson, *A Child Is Born,* Dell Publishing Company, 1990. *p. 3:* (bottom) Bonnie Kamin. *p. 4:* (left) Moredun Animal Health Ltd./Science Photo Library/Photo Researchers. (right) Biophoto Assoc./Photo Researchers/Science Source. *p. 6:* Carl Zeiss, Inc., Thornwood, New York. *p. 7:* Rockefeller Archive Center. *p. 13:* Photos by R. A. Fleischman, University of Texas, Southwestern Medical Center, Dallas. From R. A. Fleischman et al., *Proc. Natl. Acad. Sci. USA* 88:10885–10889 (1991). *pp. 20, 21, 22:* From *A Color Atlas of Histology,* S. L. Erlandsen and J. E. Magney, *Mosby Year Book, 1992.* Photo by Stan Erlandsen and Jean Magney, Dept. of Cell Biology and Neuroanatomy, University of Minnesota Medical School.

Chapter 2 *p. 24:* Pierpont Morgan Library. *p. 26:* Deutsches Museum. *p. 27:* (top left and top right) From *A Color Atlas of Histology,* S. L. Erlandsen and J. E. Magney. Photo by Stan Erlandsen and Jean Magney. (bottom left) From *A Color Atlas of Histology,* S. L. Erlandsen and J. E. Magney. Photo by Glen Giesler, Dept. of Cell Biology and Neuroanatomy, University of Minnesota Medical School. (bottom right) From *A Color Atlas of Histology,* S. L. Erlandsen and J. E. Magney. Photo by Peter Gould. *p. 29:* From *A Color Atlas of Histology,* S. L. Erlandsen and J. E. Magney. Photo by Stan Erlandsen and Jean Magney. *p. 35:* From John Cairns, *Cancer: Science and Society,* W. H. Freeman, 1978. p. 6. *p. 37:* (top) Martin M. Rotker/Photo Researchers. (center) Andrew Syred/Science Photo Library/Photo Researchers. (bottom) Robert Knauft/Photo Researchers. *p. 40:* (top) Bader/

Biological Photo Service. (bottom) Charles Albright, Whitehead Institute. *p. 41:* NIBSC/Science Photo Library/Photo Researchers. *p. 42:* Robert Pollack, Columbia University. *p. 43:* Thomas Graf et al., *Virology* 83:96–109 (1977).

Chapter 3 *p. 44:* Vincent van Gogh Foundation/Van Gogh Museum, Amsterdam. *p. 46:* Zentralbibliothek, Zurich. *p. 47:* (top) Sveriges Skorstensferjaremästares Riksförbund. (bottom) College of Physicians of Philadelphia. *p. 48:* Leiden University Library. MS Vossius lat 3, fol 90v. *p. 52:* Rockefeller Archive Center. *p. 53:* G. H. Smith, National Cancer Institute, NIH. *pp. 55, 58:* After Arnold J. Levine, *Viruses,* Scientific American Library, 1991. *p. 59:* The Granger Collection. *p. 60:* Jorge Yunis, Hahnemann University. *p. 62:* Kristien Mortelmans, SRI International, Menlo Park, Calif. *p. 63:* Bruce Ames, UC Berkeley. *p. 65:* Data from M. Meselson, Harvard University.

Chapter 4 *p. 66:* Lawrence Livermore National Laboratory. *p. 70:* Peter Vogt, University of Southern California School of Medicine. *p. 73:* From Geoffrey M. Cooper, *Oncogenes,* Jones & Bartlett, 1990. *p. 78:* Maclyn McCarty, Rockefeller University. *p. 80:* After Cooper, *Oncogenes.* *p. 81:* After J. Darnell, H. Lodish, and D. Baltimore, *Molecular Cell Biology,* 2nd ed., Scientific American Books, 1990. *p. 82:* Jorge Yunis, Hahnemann University. *p. 85:* Daniel D. Von Hoff and John McGill, University of Texas, San Antonio. Geoffrey M. Wahl, Salk Institute, La Jolla, Calif. *p. 87:* M. Baret/Rapho/Photo Researchers. *p. 88:* After Cooper, *Oncogenes.* *p. 90:* Mats Johansson and Erkki Ruoslahti. *p. 91:* (left) Mark Willingham. (right) Gilbert Jay, Red Cross Blood Labs, Rockville, Maryland. *p. 92:* After Watson et al., *Molecular Biology of the Gene,* 4th ed., Benjamin/Cummings, 1987. *p. 93:* Sung-Hou Kim, UC Berkeley. *p. 94:* After Watson et al., *Molecular Biology of the Gene.*

Chapter 5 *p. 100:* Adapted from *The Journal of NIH Research,* 1992. *p. 102:* Bernard Weissman. *p. 104:* Jorge Yunis, Hahnemann University. *p. 105:* (top) Jorge Yunis,

Hahnemann University. (bottom) Custom Medical Stock. *p. 106:* Fox Chase Cancer Center, photograph by Paul Cohen. *p. 108:* Jorge Yunis, Hahnemann University *p. 112:* Custom Medical Stock. *p. 115:* After Dr. Bert Vogelstein, Johns Hopkins University. *p. 116:* Michael English/Custom Medical Stock.

Chapter 6 *p. 120:* From W. Heath Robinson, *Inventions*, Gerald Duckworth & Co., Ltd., 1990. Colorization courtesy of *Trends in Genetics* (Elsevier Science Publishers). *p. 122:* (left) Rita Levi-Montalcini. (top right) Washington University Archives. (bottom) Stanley Cohen. *pp. 123, 128, 129:* After Darnell, Lodish, and Baltimore, *Molecular Cell Biology*. *p. 127:* Computer model done on MIDAS PLUS by Abraham de Vos and Thomas Hynes, Genentech, Inc. From A. M. de Vos, M. Ultsch, and A. A. Kossiakoff, *Science* 255:306–312. *p. 138:* (top) Vanderbilt University Archives. (bottom) Geoffrey M. Cooper, *Oncogenes*, Jones & Bartlett, 1990. *p. 140:* S. S. Taylor, J. S. Sowadski, L. Ten Eyck, and D. Knighton. From D. R. Knighton et al., *Science* 253:407–420 (1991). *p. 143:* Inder Verma, Salk Institute, La Jolla, Calif. *p. 146:* Gerald Rubin, UC Berkeley. *p. 147:* Russell J. Hill, Linda S. Huang, and Paul W. Sternberg. *p. 148:* Frank L. Margolis, Roche Institute. *p. 150:* *Scientific American*, July 1990, p. 47. *p. 151:* From A. P. McMahon, A. L. Joyner, A. Bradley, and J. A. McMahon, *Cell* 69:581–595 (1992). *p. 153:* Thomas Graf, EMBL.

Chapter 7 *p. 154:* Peter Berndt/Custom Medical Stock

Z133-FF-141 E9. *p. 157:* From John Cairns, *Cancer: Science and Society*, W. H. Freeman, 1978. *p. 161:* David Harris, Jerusalem/Archives of Weizmann, Rehovoth, Israel. *p. 164:* Philip Leder, Harvard Medical School. *p. 168:* Jorge Yunis, Hahnemann University. *p. 167:* H. Land and R. Weinberg. *p. 169:* After Levine, *Viruses*. p. 78. *p. 171:* Philip Leder, Harvard Medical School. *p. 172:* Douglas Hanahan, UC San Francisco. *p. 176:* Jorge Yunis, Hahnemann University. *p. 177:* From S. A. Rosenberg, *Scientific American* (May 1990). *p. 178:* Gilla Kaplan, The Rockefeller University. *p. 179:* (top) From Bruce Rosen et al., *Magnetic Resonance in Medicine* 19 (1991). (bottom) Judah Folkman, Children's Hospital, Harvard Medical School. *p. 180:* Lance A. Liotta. *p. 182:* After L. A. Liotta, *Scientific American* (February 1992). *p. 183:* Garth Nicolson.

Chapter 8 *p. 187:* Adapted from Mark Leppert, Dept. of Genetics, University of Utah. *p. 189:* After Darnell, Lodish, and Baltimore, *Molecular Cell Biology*. *pp. 190, 191:* From Cairns, *Cancer: Science and Society*. *p. 192:* Electron Microscopy Laboratory, The Lindsley F. Kimball Research Institute, A Division of the New York Blood Center. *p. 193:* Institut de Virologie, Tours, France. *p. 194:* (left) Cabisco/Visuals Unlimited. (right) Custom Medical Stock. *p. 195:* Visuals Unlimited. *p. 196:* After K. B. Mullis, *Scientific American*, (April 1990). *p. 198:* Harold Varmus. *p. 199:* James Prince/Photo Researchers. *pp. 204, 205:* After I. M. Verma, *Scientific American* (November 1990). *p. 206:* Helen Coley Nauts.

Index

SUGGESTIONS FOR FURTHER READING

Brugge, J., T. Curran, E. Harlow, and F. McCormick, eds. *Origins of Human Cancer*. Cold Spring Harbor Laboratory, 1991.

Cairns, J. *Cancer: Science and Society*. San Francisco: W. H. Freeman, 1978.

Cooper, G. M. *Oncogenes*. Boston: Jones and Bartlett, 1990.

Franks, L. M., and N. Teich. *Introduction to the Cellular and Molecular Biology of Cancer*. New York: Oxford University Press, 1986.

Friedberg, E. C., ed. *Cancer Biology: Readings from Scientific American*. New York: W. H. Freeman, 1986.

Gross, L. *Oncogenic Viruses*. 3d ed. Elmsford, N.Y.: Pergamon Press, 1983.

Tannock, I. F., and R. P. Hill. *The Basic Science of Oncology*. Elmsford, N.Y.: Pergamon Press, 1987.

Varmus, H., and A. J. Levine, eds. *Readings in Tumor Virology*. Cold Spring Harbor Laboratory, 1983.

Weinberg, R. A., ed. *Oncogenes and the Molecular Origins of Cancer*. Cold Spring Harbor Laboratory, 1990.